T0271968

Routledge Revivals

The limbo people

First published in 1980, *The limbo people* is based upon research carried out in a day centre ('the Centre') for elderly Jewish people in a London Borough and studies the experience and the conception of time among the elderly. The development of the arguments concerning time was founded on (a) the relationship between the community of participants and the outside world; and (b) the construction of events and interactions between participants at the Centre. The organization of this book re-enacts the process of reconstituting time as manifested in the Centre, against the background of the participants previous experiences, and in terms of their present existential situations. This book will be of interest to students of sociology, anthropology and gerontology.

The limbo people

A study of the constitution of the time universe
among the aged

Haim Hazan

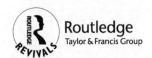

Routledge
Taylor & Francis Group

First published in 1980
By Routledge & Kegan Paul Ltd

This edition first published in 2023 by Routledge
4 Park Square, Milton Park, Abingdon, Oxon, OX14 4RN
and by Routledge
605 Third Avenue, New York, NY 10017

Routledge is an imprint of the Taylor & Francis Group, an informa business

Publisher's Note
The publisher has gone to great lengths to ensure the quality of this reprint but points
out that some imperfections in the original copies may be apparent.

Disclaimer
The publisher has made every effort to trace copyright holders and welcomes
correspondence from those they have been unable to contact.

A Library of Congress record exists under ISBN: 0710004818

ISBN: 978-1-032-49974-1 (hbk)
ISBN: 978-1-003-39631-4 (ebk)
ISBN: 978-1-032-49977-2 (pbk)

Book DOI 10.4324/9781003396314

The limbo people

A study of the constitution of the time universe among the aged

Haim Hazan

Department of Sociology and Anthropology
University of Tel-Aviv

Routledge & Kegan Paul

London, Boston and Henley

To Mercia

First published in 1980
by Routledge & Kegan Paul Ltd
39 Store Street, London WC1E 7DD,
Broadway House, Newtown Road,
Henley-on-Thames, Oxon RG9 1EN and
9 Park Street, Boston, Mass. 02108, USA
Set in 10 on 12pt English Times
and printed in Great Britain by
Thomson Litho Ltd, East Kilbride, Scotland

Set by Colset Pte Ltd
Singapore

British Library Cataloguing in Publication Data

Hazan, Haim

The limbo people. — (International library of
anthropology).
1. Old age assistance — England — London
metropolitan area — Case studies
2. Jewish aged — England — London metropolitan
area — Case studies 3. Community health services
for the aged — England — London metropolitan area
— Case studies 4. Time perception — Case studies
I. Title II. Series
362.6'11'2   HV1481.G5   79-42732

ISBN 0 7100 0481 8

Contents

Tables

Acknowledgments

The research would not have been possible without the co-operation, the understanding and the very amicable attitude towards me by both participants and staff. The warm reception and the unconditional acceptance I enjoyed made an invaluable contribution to the study.

I am particularly grateful for the active interest in the research shown by the supervisor of the Centre and his team, an attitude which apart from personal encouragement was manifested in free access to staff meetings, documentation and other various sources of information.

In analysing and organizing the data, I would like to express my gratitude to Dr M. Gilsenan, my supervisor, whose guidance and advice throughout my studies were of great assistance to me.

I would also like to express my thanks to Professor A. Kuper for his interest in the research and his encouragement.

My approach in this research has been much influenced by Professor M. Douglas's work and this, in addition to the personal interest she has extended to me, has proven to be an invaluable source of inspiration.

Many useful remarks and pieces of advice came from members of the Department of Sociology and Anthropology in Tel-Aviv University. I am particularly grateful to Professor E. Marx whose insight was of great help to me in developing a theoretical perspective on the ethnography.

The financial support I received throughout the fieldwork from Tel-Aviv University and the Memorial Foundation for Jewish Culture (NY) was essential to the completion of the research.

The study could not have been accomplished without the dedicated effort of my wife, Mercia, who spent countless hours deciphering the manuscript, typing it and adding her valuable comments.

The index was compiled by Richard Raper.

Haim Hazan

Introduction: The emergence of the time factor

The research upon which this book is based was carried out in a day centre ('the Centre') for elderly Jewish people in a London Borough. My encounter with the social world of the members of the establishment (the 'participants', as they were referred to by themselves and by members of the staff), provoked a whole gamut of sociological questions, but I gradually recognized the supreme importance of their preoccupation with the management of time. Although this discovery was made at rather a late stage of the field-work, it was in many ways a sequel to previously developed perspectives on the Centre reality, as well as a new avenue for its exploration. The path to this recognition may be briefly indicated.

First, encounters with participants quickly suggested a division into two major categories: those who professed to use the Centre merely for its material provisions, as a day shelter and communal kitchen, and those who declared that for them the meaning of the Centre extended far beyond the obvious services it provided. The former group tended to view the Centre as a transitional, insignificant stage in their lives, divorced from their outside world, while for the latter the Centre was the hub, the most meaningful part of their existence.

This differentiation between Centre-oriented participants and the others, more attached to the outside world, corresponded closely to the length of attendance at the Centre. Thus 'new arrivals' expressed less commitment to a Centre-oriented life than did the veterans. Furthermore, an unmistakable and consistent change of attitude was noticeable among one-time newcomers who began to attend the Centre regularly. They seemed to have undergone a process of conversion into full commitment to the Centre world. Consequently, instead of concentrating on superficially clear-cut distinctions, the research was diverted into an examination of some of the characteristics which marked the transition from mere attendance to participation.

In the course of examining the nature of the transformation, and the content of the relationship between 'instructors' and 'novices', it became clear that most of the interactions between participants were governed by a code of behaviour and attitudes which stressed the paramount importance of care and help. This recurrent theme, when analysed and linked with other aspects of the Centre reality, revealed certain fundamental differences between the system of exchange in the Centre and the nature of reciprocal relationships in the outside world. The main differences involved contrasting attitudes towards personal life history, present conditions, and future prospects. The importance of time perspective and time experience began to be clear. The structure of events, and inter-action among participants, particularly when contrasted with the organization of life in the period preceding Centre attendance, also began to make better sense once the temporal dimension was granted analytical significance.

In unravelling the time universe of the Centre people I used an empirical approach, but had to grapple with a highly abstract concept of time. The literature, though extensive, was of limited value to me, since in general it treated time as a reflection of other social determinants, while the change undergone by the partici-pants demanded an understanding of time as something to be mani-pulated and reconstructed. Although I was helped by a few writers who analysed time as a resource, I concluded that an appropriate definition must be sought in the fieldwork material, and emerge from the Centre reality itself. Thus the development of the argu-ments concerning time was founded on (a) the relationship between the community of participants and the outside world; and (b) the construction of events and interactions between participants at the Centre. The organization of this book re-enacts the process of reconstituting time as manifested in the Centre, against the back-ground of the participants' previous experiences, and in terms of their present existential situation.

The first chapter deals with the various social determinants of the pre-Centre situation, particularly with its incongruities and ambiguities. This is followed by an analysis of the Centre as an isolated haven, sequestered from the outside world. The third chapter discusses the views and attitudes of participants towards their past and their future, and the fourth chapter concentrates on the construction of the social reality in the Centre, with special attention directed to the implications of the relationship between participants for their conception of time. The last part of the book describes the social structure of the Centre, in relation to the temporal dimension ingrained in it. This discussion is complemented by an account of the system of social control developed in the Centre, and the process of participation, from initiation into the society of the Centre to membership of divisions within it.

1   The limbo state

For most participants, entering the Centre means not only a new start, but a milestone on the path along which they have been passing in recent years. The period preceding the Centre is essential to the understanding of the reality in the Centre and, therefore, special attention should be paid to its exploration.

Getting old is for the Centre population[1] a span of their life cycle dominated by two interwoven determinants. The first is the emergence of some gradual changes in physical condition and mental state, coupled with inescapable personal crises, such as a death in the family, illness, etc. The second is the encounter with social environment which provides them with some basic needs whilst alienating them from any meaningful involvement. This combination of personal plight and social impoverishment presents a situation in which no restoration of the past is conceivable, no progress towards new goals feasible. The unravelling of the various facets of this limbo state and the examination of the existential implications of its impact on the people entering the Centre will be the subject of this chapter.

The main course of the discussion and hence the structure of the following sections is based on the assumption that the process of growing old could be characterized by a fundamental incongruity between some aspects of the social definition of old people and their place in society and the actual experience of unarrested deterioration in later life. This incompatibility, being the cardinal source for some significant changes in the time perspectives of the elderly, requires examination both diachronically and synchronically.

Pre-Centre situations could be divided into four analytical areas of concern which also delineate the structure of the chapter. The first concerns the socio-economic history of the participants, from childhood to their situation preceding their admission to the

Centre. This is followed by a description of the everyday difficulties caused by illness and bereavement. The third section will discuss general social attitudes encountered by the elderly. In the fourth section we arrive at the decision-making process which eventually leads to entering the Centre.

Disintegration

The Centre, being designated to serve and cater for Jewish people in the north-east of London, recruits the great bulk of its participants from the Jewish population of the London Borough of Marlsden. This is an amalgamation of several former metropolitan boroughs carried out in 1965 in, implementation of the Local Government Act 1963, which provided for reorganization of local government in the London area. It has a population of 219,240 in an area of 4,814 acres.

As an individual area, the borough has absorbed a large number of immigrants who have taken over jobs and accommodation vacated by the ageing or the population who have moved away. This has created a multi-racial multi-ethnic community of which the Jews comprise the largest minority, numbering 30,360 (data applicable to 1971).[2] The second largest minority, the West Indians, number only 16,830.

Between the turn of the century and the early 1950s the Jewish population of the borough rose whilst the general population sharply declined (from 389,000 in 1901 to 265,000 in 1951). Towards the 1960s and later on, this trend was arrested and as a result of migration processes, the Jewish population gradually decreased and changed its age structure and socio-economic characteristics.[3]

> The Jewish population pyramid reveals that few of the offspring of persons over the age of 54 remained in the Borough when they married since there is a marked under-representation of persons aged 24 – 54. This has produced an aged population. The meridian for the Jewish population is 42 years which is 6 years more than for the general population at 36 years. Because of this ageing the Jewish population has a female sex bias.

As the purpose of this study is not a demographic analysis of the overall Jewish population of Marlsden, the discussion will be limited to the impact of some general trends and processes as manifested in the composition of the Centre population. The present characteristics of these people are, therefore, a starting point for a biographical inquiry and in particular exploration of the last stage of their life cycle.

There are three shared groups of factors in these people's lives which might be seen as main lines underpinning their individual biographies and, hence, allow us to adopt a generalized perspective on their past. The first relates to changes in the family, the second concerns their socio-economic positions and the third their place within the Jewish community, particularly with regard to their involvement with the activities of the Jewish Welfare Board. Their lives could be divided, approximately, into three consecutive phases marked off from each other by some fundamental changes in these three factors. Starting as immigrants, children and young adults, in the East End of London, they resettled in Marlsden, and now find themselves in their present situation of dependency, desertion and disintegration.[4]

'Since the very beginning of the industrial revolution, the East End has provided a kind of unofficial "reception centre" for a succession of immigrant communities in flight from religious persecution or economic depression' (Cohen, 1972, p.9). Following the anti-Semitic measures introduced in Russia during the 1880s a constant flow of Jewish refugees landed in England, some of them having been stranded on their way to America with no money to continue their journey, and settled mostly in that 'reception centre' of the East End. Restricted by language difficulties and discriminated against by the other inhabitants of the East End, and in particular by the existing well-established Jewish community, the newcomers found themselves with no means for essential sustenance. Jobs were scarce as a result of a general trade depression and support from relatives was by no means a sufficient and stable basis for living (Wischnitzer, 1948, ch. III). Under these circumstances the only way of seeking help was to apply to the Jewish Welfare Board, known at that time as the Jewish Board of Guardians.

The Jewish Welfare Board is a charitable organization founded in 1859 by representatives of the three main London synagogues for the relief of the poor immigrant Jews — 'strange poor' as they used to be called — who were not eligible for the assistance of the

organized Jewish community. The intents of the new body covered
(1) relief — e.g. jobs and apprenticeship schemes, (2) temporary
allowances, (3) fixed allowances, (4) emigration, i.e. inducing
repatriation of clients, and (5) clothing and coal (Magnus, 1909,
p.39).

Eligibility of an applicant was assessed by an 'investigating
officer' who carried out a thoroughly detailed means test which was
passed on to various committees. The activities of the Board
expanded considerably in response to the growing need for assistance caused by increased immigration and worsening economic
conditions in the East End (Lipman, 1959, chs IV, V).

Most of the parents of Day Centre participants were at one time
or another amongst the beneficiaries of the Board's services, and
whilst not on the dole, they were engaged in unskilled or semi-
skilled occupations particularly in the tailoring and the furniture
industries and also as hawkers, street traders, etc. The Board's
penetration into the family by employment and apprenticeship
schemes made the second generation well aware of its presence.

The close-knit matrilocal kinship network in the East End, being
the major feature of family ties amongst the Jewish community of
the area, provided a supportive system of care based on mutual
multiplex obligations. This interlocking pattern linking several
families was an integral part of the wider arena of community life.
People knew each other and were involved socially, politically and
economically in an integrated, almost self-sufficient working-class
community.

The ecology of the district with its narrow streets, back-to-back
terraced houses, corner shops and small workshops attached to
residences, facilitated neighbourliness and daily interaction which
was intensive and frequent. This together with proliferating congre-
gational establishments like synagogues, schools, public baths,
local charities, etc. accentuated and furnished the atmosphere of
solidarity and cohesiveness.

Although the relation of this description to the reality of life in
the East End during the first decades of the century might not be
factually established, it is nevertheless the picture disseminated by
the participants in the Centre and as such represents their concept,
perhaps an embellished, nostalgic one, of their childhood and early
adulthood. As their lives at present stand in a self-conceived sharp
contrast to that past, this biased concept is significant to the main

changes in their lives.

A tendency for well-to-do East End families to move out, north-bound, became increasingly noticeable towards the 1930s, and was accelerated as a result of the Second World War. The East End being a main target for German air raids on London, was severely affected by the war. Families lost their accommodation and as a result were evacuated to the suburbs or the country. After the war was over, they had nowhere to return to and consequently they were resettled in neighbouring districts, particularly in Marlsden where there was already an established Jewish community with a large number of former East Enders.

The boom in employment which followed the war reduced considerably the number of able-bodied applicants to the Board. This, coupled with the introduction of statutory social legislation overlapping the Board's services, changed the traditional clientele of the Board from the unemployed, the disabled and the widows to European war refugees and the evacuees. The present aged population of Marlsden was fully employed rearing young families and in no need of charitable assistance. Community institutions were flourishing and flows of orthodox Jewish east European immigrants settled in the area made for a mixed, segmentary Jewish community.

Religiously a wide spectrum of western Jewry was represented, ranging from the extremely isolated, self-contained sect of 'Naturei Karta', to middle-of-the-road Jews still belonging to synagogues and holding on to certain aspects of the traditional Jewish way of life as experienced by them in their childhood, to self-confessed non-believers who seem to have dissociated themselves from any vestige of religion. These groups vary considerably in the degree of integration with the non-Jewish population in their cultural orientation and background and in the type of social relationship within each section. This created some insuperable barriers between different groups of Jews in the area both socially and ecologically.

The range of trades and occupations had not changed significantly, but the former system of an interlocked source of subsistence, residence, friendships and political conviction no longer operated. The nuclear family had become the predominant pattern of kinship, and life revolved mainly around the axis of the relationship between parents and children with diminishing emphasis on involvement in community activities.

Around the 1960s the dwindling of the Jewish population in the area had reached its climax. It was due to the combined effect of two phenomena both stemming from one demographic determinant. The post-war prosperity brought about a move of a large number of families from Marlsden to the new core of Jewish life in London – the north-west. There was a steady flow of the comfortably-off, self-employed and professionals, who joined the already existing affluent Jewish communities of Golders Green, Hampstead and Hendon. They were joined later by younger families composed mainly of the children of those who moved to Marlsden. The majority of those who could not afford to make their way to the north-west have also left the area and settled in other districts far away from their parents.

The gap between the third generation of well-assimilated, well-educated children and the socially uprooted, hard-up generation of their parents could be illustrated by the following figures. All the data are based on information obtained from the participants of the Centre and from their records in the Jewish Welfare Board's archives and refer to 280 participants.

TABLE 1.1 *Number of children and marital status (in percentages)*

Marital status	Number of children		
	1	*2 – 3*	*4 +*
Married couples	29	13.2	0.6
Previously married or separated	38.4	17.6	1.2

The high percentage of single child families gives some grounds for the allegation of desertion and negligence made by the elderly. This allegation was less noticeable in families with more than one child for there was a greater probability of care and concern shown by some of the children. This care and concern sociologically manifests itself in two complementary forms: contact and financial support. As it was not technically feasible to extract adequate relevant information and assessments from the children concerned, it was inevitably necessary to rely mainly on the parents' evaluation, combined with reports by social workers who invariably sided with their clients and thus confirmed the parents' point of view. It should be noted, however, that in the course of the fieldwork and as a result of establishing a trust relationship with some of the participants, it has become apparent that there is a considerable incongruity between these subjective estimations and the actual situation. This is to say that in effect children do visit, contact and support their parents more than the latter are willing to admit.

Researchers such as Townsend (1973) and Johnson (1975) remarked on the inconsistency between the social conception of the generation gap and reality. In our case this gap is evidently promoted by the picture constructed by the aged themselves. The reasons behind this misrepresentation varied from sheer economic considerations − buttressing an application for financial aid − to a confessed desire to minimize the effect of such existing, wavering, tantalizing links as occasional phone calls, sporadic visits divorced from real participation and influence in the family life. The sorest point is the inability to maintain regular and frequent contact with the grandchildren − a painful disengagement which was a source of constant aggravation and regret to the grandparents.

Any statistical measurement of support, let alone contact, is highly unreliable and, therefore, unsatisfactory and, in view of the above reservations, it is particularly difficult in this case. Nevertheless, acceptable criteria such as number of visits, regularity and conceived intensity of relationships could be employed to give a rough assessment of these variables. According to this, the relative contact maintained between parents and their children, taken mainly from the formers' point of view, is as in Table 1.2.

TABLE 1.2 *Number of children maintaining contact with parents according to parents' marital status (in percentages)*

Marital status	Degree of contact		
	Regular	Occasional	None
Married couples	13.4	15.2	18.3
Previously married and separated	27.0	10.4	15.7

It is evident that the perceived social isolation of married couples is far greater than that of the previously married (mainly widows). It is also conspicuous that over 30 per cent of the children are alleged to have no contact whatsoever with their parents and this receives an added dimension from the data related to material support as shown in Table 1.3.

TABLE 1.3 *Number of children supporting their parents according to parents' marital status (in percentages)*

Marital status	Support		
	Regular	*Occasional*	*None*
Married couples	0.1	2.5	26.6
Previously married	1.1	1.2	68.5

The negligible number of children rendering regular or even occasional support to their parents corroborates the assumption that one of the reasons for parents consciously disengaging themselves from their children is the realization that their concern and interest in their offspring is too often ignored, and reciprocal relationships fail to develop. In this respect the predicament of widows and widowers is far graver, for they maintain a higher degree of regular contact, but at the same time, being unable to lean on a spouse, are deprived of a comparable support.

The predicament would have been avoided had the children been unable to help, but as things stand there is little question as to their resources. The popular saying amongst Marlsden Jews that the distance between the East End and Golders Green is two generations, relates mainly to the difference in status and class. Geographical and social distance make some of these children virtually unreachable by their parents. Remarks such as 'I cannot go there because all their friends are so educated and well-spoken and they will be ashamed of me' are fairly common amongst the participants and clearly indicate the barrier of conceived inferiority which interferes with any attempt to tighten the relationship. Tables 1.4, 1.5 and 1.6 refer to the factors of geographical and social distance:

TABLE 1.4 *Number of children according to areas of residence and parents' marital status (in percentages)*

Marital status	Area of residence		
	Marlsden*	*Suburbs***	*Outside London****
Married couples	0.9	37	7
Previously married	4.7	39	11.4

*   Most of the children living in Marlsden are unmarried looking after their parents or in some cases of mental disorder or retardation looked after by the parents.

** Including the West End and Ilford.

***Including children living abroad.

The limbo state

TABLE 1.5 *Proportion of children according to occupation and parents' marital status (in percentages)*

Marital status	Occupation		
	Professionals and skilled*	Semi- and non-skilled**	Not working***
Married couples	29	10	3.7
Previously married and separated	36	18	3.3

* Occupations requiring special qualifications or training.

** Manual jobs and casual trades.

***Daughters who are housewives were categorized according to their husband's occupation so that this category refers mostly to the unemployed.

TABLE 1.6 *Occupation of parents and year of retirement in relation to date of entering the Centre (in percentages — non working males and females were eliminated)*

Year of retirement	Occupation			
	Professional and semi-skilled		Unskilled	
	Males	Females	Males	Females
Retired within one year	1.5	0.1	29	0.1
Retired within five years	1.2	–	50.5	0.4
Retired over five years	0.5	0.2	15.6	0.9

The very high proportion of unskilled parents affects not only the relationship between them and their children, but also to the place taken by work amongst other aspects of their lives. Most of the trades held by these people offered no career in the sense of professional progress and profit-making, nor did they suggest special satisfaction or sense of achievement. In fact, most of the participants spoke of their working life as a compelling, unpleasant, tedious, necessary evil and hence regarded their retirement as a welcome relief.

Needless to say, most of these unskilled occupations provided no adequate financial security for old age and, therefore, the only means available to combat impending poverty is by using statutory and other public entitlements. Hence, the profile of the participants' weekly income compositions is as shown in Table 1.7.

Over one-third of the participants are forced to live only off their retirement state pension and another 40 per cent enjoy supplementary benefits. Hence, apart from 11.5 per cent who have some

TABLE 1.7 *Composition of weekly income (in percentages)*

SS	PR	OP	PR+OP	PR+SS	PR+OP +SS	PR+OP+ SS+CH	CH+SS	CH+SS +OP	OP+SS	Only SP	Total
40	1	2	1	9	1	0.5	1	0.3	8.7	36.5	100

SP = State Pension; SS = Social Security (supplementary benefits, etc.); CH = Childrens' Support; OP = Other Pensions (war pension, work, etc.); PR = Private Means (savings, property, etc.)

Note: This table is based on the fact that over 90 per cent of the participants receive SP. Also, logical combinations such as PR + CH or PR + OP + CH which do not apply to any of the participants were eliminated from the table.

private resources (mainly savings amounting to a few hundred pounds) and 13.5 per cent who receive other pensions, the majority of participants have a fixed very limited weekly income which merely enables them to pay for the bare essentials of existence like food and heating. Anything beyond that is unobtainable. Thus a single person living on his own and being in receipt of a state pension plus social security constituting a weekly income of approximately £15 can just about manage to cover the expenses of rent, electricity, gas, heating, basic food and some other bare essentials. Being faced with a sharp rise in the cost of living unmatched by a corresponding increase in income, most of the elderly experienced a gradual deterioration in their standard of living.

In order to maintain a desirable standard of living, many people take advantage of public services available to the aged. There are two main facilities which are highly utilized by the elderly and which contribute considerably to the alleviation of their financial and physical difficulties. One is the Meals on Wheels service, or alternatively, the Kosher Meals on Wheels charity which provides the elderly with a cheap, hot, nourishing meal a day in their own residence. The other is the range of services offered by local authorities such as home help, charladies to clean, district nurse, mobile libraries, installation of special facilities such as bath rails, etc. There are, of course, a number of charities and other organizations catering for specific needs for selected sectors of the population.

Evidently there is an under-utilization of services and there is an incompatibility between high need and low demand. Some of the reasons for this will be discussed further on, but it should be noted that self-imposed social isolation following bereavement is one of the main impediments in searching for means of mitigating hard-

TABLE 1.8 *People using public facilities according to their marital status (in percentages)*

Marital status	Facilities and services					
	KMOW	LAS	O	KMOW+LAS	LAS+O	None
Married	3.6	7	–	–	3	15
Widows and widowers	–	30.4	1.3	1.1	4	28
Unmarried, divorced and separated	–	1.6	–	–	–	5

KMOW = Kosher Meals on Wheels; LAS = Local Authority Services; O = Other services and facilities.

ships. Around 50 per cent of the Centre population are people who have suffered a recent loss of a spouse, and are in a state of bereavement. This trying period of loneliness and depression has clinched for most of them the realization that they have been deserted by their children. The few polite visits and occasional phone calls made by the children created a final insuperable barrier between them and their parents. The feeling of being forsaken by their children coupled by lack of support from other kith and kin accentuate considerably the conceived reality of a dismembered family and alienated society. This wilful isolation ramifies into other areas of relationships between the aged individual and his social environment. It particularly affects participation and involvement in activities available or especially designed for the elderly. There are numerous clubs, day centres, workshops for the elderly, etc. scattered all over the area offering company, interest, and even money to participants, yet as shown in table 1.9 these services are also barely taken advantage of.

TABLE 1.9 *People attending clubs etc. according to marital status (in percentages)*

Marital status	Facilities										
	C	D	S	O	C+D	C+D+S	C+S	C+O	D+S	D+O+S	None
Married	–	0.2	3.7	3	–	–	0.3	–	–	–	5
Widows and widowers	5	–	20	0.2	0.7	1.1	0.1	1.8	1	8	40.5
Unmarried, divorced and separated	4	3.3	0.1	0.9	–	–	0.7	–	–	–	0.4

C = Social clubs, friendship clubs; D = Day centres (apart from the one in question; S = Synagogues; O = Others such as workshops for the elderly and luncheon clubs

Most of the members of the synagogues do not attend regularly, but pay the membership fees to ensure Jewish burial arrangements for themselves. Unmarried people are more outgoing than bereaved people. This may be accounted for by the undisrupted continuation of former activities, in contrast to the breakdown in social life experienced by widows and widowers. In this respect, married people occupy an intermediate position, for they can still maintain their relationship with their social environment, with the poignant exclusion of their children.

One of the very few stable, long-standing, fundamentally unchanged factors in this social environment is the presence of the Jewish Welfare Board. Most of the people concerned, having been acquainted with its activities through their parents' plight or their own problems, know of its purposes and services and have some image of the expected pattern of relationship between the organiza-tion and its clients. This image, of nineteenth-century patronizing charity, has deterred quite a number of eligible elderly people from applying to the Board for help, but there was a deeper inhibition which made people reluctant to consider the Board's assistance.

The Jewish Welfare Board is traditionally associated with the first staggering steps of an East End generation of eastern Euro-pean refugees, unskilled, ignorant of the language and alien to the culture − the participants' parents. This association brings shame and indignity on those who have still remained under the auspices of this organization. Furthermore, by being confronted with their well-to-do East End contemporaries in affluent suburbia − many of them donors to the Jewish Welfare Board − potential applicants are presented with a grave dilemma. Applying to the organization for help plunges them into an area of stigma and humiliation emphasizing the lack of progress they have made in relation to their parents and in contrast to their friends. Yet although refraining from applying for the Board's services might spare one the unpleasant connotations involved, it would leave few resources available to combat hardship.

The temptation to apply should not be underestimated. The Jewish Welfare Board offers a range of various allowances, well-equipped modern old age homes, supportive social workers' visits, etc. and for people who are in need of all this, it is rather hard to resist. What makes up people's minds one way or the other is a combination of four variables; family intervention, ability to cope with deteriorating health and increasing loneliness, state of mind and general outlook on life, and the existence of alternatives.

Coping

The first encounter with members of the helping professions usually occurs against the background of a disintegrated community and a dismembered family. A person is struck by the realization that he can no longer cope with his life as it is and some form of assistance should be sought. The point at which this realization is reached is by no means a unitary one and in most cases it indicates a stage in a long, fluctuating process of deterioration. The relative ability of different people to sustain the pressure of their worsening conditions makes it virtually meaningless sharply to distinguish between a 'coping with' syndrome and a 'giving up' situation. However, certain strains and imbalances are germane to the process as a whole and, therefore, might shed some light on the characteristics of the pre-Centre situation.

A viable starting point could be the views of the people from whom help is normally sought. Social workers' assessments of clients seldom fail to note 'unable to cope' and 'ill health'. One attribute without the other is regarded as anomalous. Thus a client living in a bedsitter and applying for better accommodation is described thus in a report: 'Tends to groan and acts as a very ill woman, although she is self-sufficient'; and indeed very few clients who suffer from ill health give the impression of being able to look after themselves properly.

Illness in old age differs from most illnesses inflicted on younger people in a few respects. Most are chronic diseases with rather bleak prognoses and, unlike other ailments which are temporary, they are likely to accompany the old person with low resistance for the rest of his life. Another common condition is the fact that old people are usually afflicted by more than one disease either simultaneously or within very short intervals. Thus it would be rather difficult to point to a certain ailment to specify the particular hardships it entails and to forecast the future.

'Suffers from angina, hiatus hernia and kidney troubles.'

'Mrs M. has had both breasts removed, her legs are extremely swollen and she suffers from high blood pressure. She also has cataracts and has recently become slightly deaf.'

These quotations from social workers' reports represent a general indicator of the health of the old people applying for social services and such assessments could be completed by the accounts given by the elderly themselves.[5]

> I am fine
> There is nothing whatever the matter with me
> I am just as healthy as can be;
> I have arthritis in both my knees
> And when I talk, I talk with a wheeze!
> My pulse is weak and my blood is thin!
> But I'm awfully well for the shape I'm in.
>
> I think my liver is out of whack
> And I've a terrible pain in my back
> My hearing's poor, and my eyes are dim
> Most everything seems to be out of trim
> The way I stagger sure is a crime
> I'm likely to fall most any time:
> But all things considered, I'm feeling fine!
>
> Now the moral is, as this tale I unfold
> That for you and me who are growing old
> It's better to say 'I'm fine' with a grin
> Than to tell everyone the shape we are in!

The attitude of ironical acceptance and pretence in the face of an unsurmountable assemblage of ailments can smooth out one's social interaction with non-ailing people, but does not, and indeed is not, designed to alleviate the implied daily difficulties one has to cope with.

Considering the number of illnesses, ranging from mild attacks of arthritis to terminal cancer, from which old people suffer, it would be pointless to typify their multiplexity by tables and patterns. Instead we would try to trace some of the implications caused by diseases and the way they pervade almost every aspect of the elderly person's life.

Whatever the pre-disease daily routine of a person might have been, it is bound to be severely disrupted by regular visits to hospitals for check-ups and treatment. A great number of Centre applicants are out-patients who have recently been hospitalized for some time. This requires regular journeys followed by long waiting hours in the hospital and as most of them are handicapped to a certain extent, the whole outing takes time as much as energy so that long preparations and proper rest are often needed. On top of this, there are always the frequent visits to the local doctor and the constant vigilance required to control the ever-changing intake of drugs, which together make an old person's medical condition very much a new integral part of his life, governing his daily routine.

The nature of the disease may also play a dominant role in altering one's environmental boundaries. Crippling diseases such as rheumatoid arthritis and osteoarthritis delimit considerably one's mobility and may curtail significantly the ability to move about and to go out for shopping or recreation. In severe cases people become practically housebound and the effects of this could be detrimental to their already deteriorating general physical and mental state. With the absence of a regular home-help people experience increasing difficulties in performing the daily chores around the house and, as shopping is too much of a hardship, some of them are forced to live on an unnourishing uncooked diet of tinned food, accompanied by quite often bad or, in some cases, non-existent heating, and squalid surroundings. In social workers' reports one can find remarks like 'Mr E. looks more like a wild animal at bay'; or 'He won't wash or change and looks filthy.'

Indeed, many of the housebound are aided by sticks, crutches, walking frames and wheelchairs, but the process of getting used to such stigmatizing aids is a trying, often painful ordeal which leaves its traces in the form of further isolation and withdrawal.

In every disease there is an element of uncertainty and as a rule the greater the uncertainty the more obsessed with it the sick person becomes. People learn rather fast how to tackle their new daily-limited physical world, but the anxieties, the fear and the perplexity caused by an unpredictable course of illness is more difficult to cope with. Past experience proves to be useless in encountering the new situation and plans for the future have to be abandoned. Doctors' advice and explanations, if given at all, are received with mistrust and provide neither comfort nor reassurance.

Two examples of the response to incurable diseases could demonstrate the effect of uncertainty and fear on the patient's life. A fifty-three-year-old man suffering from multiple sclerosis was told by his doctor that his brain was functioning 'like the brain of a seventy-year-old' and it would be advisable for him to refrain from being engaged in any strenuous activity requiring excessive mental effort. As the course of this degenerative disease included intermittent remissions and relapses, the man was incapable of assessing either his mental ability or his physical fitness. His resources and potentialities became as obscure as the disease itself and constant confusion and frustration have taken the place of a well-planned life.

Haunted by the overwhelming effect of the disease, he tried desperately to reorientate himself by gaining more than a layman's knowledge of the nature of his affliction. This he hoped to achieve by scanning medical magazines, looking at casual medical books and eagerly listening to other patients' experiences. Needless to say, this was doomed to failure. His attempts have brought him more distress and confusion than before. Consequently, he looked no more for panaceas or for temporary relief, all his attention now being directed to learning ways of coping with his immediate environment, solving problems which ranged from climbing stairs to securing his welfare benefits.

Another man suffering from a heart condition, severe diabetes, kidney disorders and cancer of the throat had unsurprisingly found himself rather puzzled by the interwoven symptoms and varied treatments. Having given up any attempt to disentangle his medical muddle, he developed a fervent interest in showing other people how he had learnt to cope with the daily difficulties caused by the various effects of his ailments.

This increased contraction of one's world to the daily present confrontation with difficulties imposed by ill health not only forestalls any plans for the future, but also involves a realization that some highly significant elements from one's past are never to be restored. Thus a hard-of-hearing musician was forced to give up his profession as well as his fulfilling hobby. A local politician found himself unable to attend meetings and committees and consequently was compelled to retire. A prostate operation resulting in impotency severely curtailed another person's ability to lead an intensive sex life as he alleged he had been used to do. All in all, a gap has been created between one's desires, habits and range of significance, and the diminishing ability to keep all those things within reach.

The damage to a person's self-image is sometimes far worse than the actual deprivation imposed by the disease. It may alter completely a person's conception of his situation as a human being and his position in relation to other people. A few people even said that they no longer regarded themselves as human beings. Their engrossment with their physical condition did not allow them to claim that title. The analysis of the concept of human being prevailing amongst these people is beyond the scope of this discussion, but it is worth noting that their judgments here are marked by the association between the feeling of uselessness, unworthiness and frustration, and a conviction about time, namely the irreversibility of the past coupled with the unpredictability of the future.

The intensity of this self-degradation is not determined merely by the disease itself and the nature of the loss incurred by it. There are some significant differences between the reactions of people who are afflicted by the same illness and suffer similar losses. One major factor here is the effect of the illness on the relationship with other people especially between spouses, and particularly on the division of labour within the family and the conjugal roles of husband and wife.

As is common among working-class people of their generation, most of the elderly couples were used to a rather strict domestic division of labour. The husband was the bread-winner, and the wife was in charge of housekeeping and rearing the children. Retirement and illness might bring about an upheaval in this situation which could take one of two contrary forms.

The first is when a husband is no longer capable of providing for his family whereas his wife is still fit enough to go out to work and to sustain them both. Apart from the indignity and humiliation endured by the husband, the whole structure of power between the couple is altered. A stage may come when a wife decides to get her husband into an old age home or a geriatric ward. This might happen when the conflicting demands of looking after a sick husband, keeping a house and earning a living can no longer be sustained by the wife. Arriving at such a decision often indicates a total breakdown of trust relationships and loyalties built over the years of married life. As a social worker described one of his cases:

> 'Mrs G. raised these matters (of making an old age home application on behalf of her husband) in hushed tones before I met her husband, and obviously he is not himself aware that his wife may be trying to get him placed in a Home. He would be told

that it was for an extended holiday since he might otherwise object to the arrangement.'

A much more common situation is that in which the husband takes the responsibility for the housekeeping as well as the daily care of his ill wife. The following description taken from a social worker's report exemplifies what might happen in that event:

'Mr P. is sixty years old and is still working as a furniture fitter. He leaves home at 7 a.m. and only returns normally at 7 p.m. Before leaving he gets his wife up and dresses her and gives her breakfast, but she usually lies down again after he has gone out of the house. When he comes home at night he makes the coal fire and then gets supper for himself and his wife. He shops at week-ends and seems to be very capable around the house ... . He has to be very careful about turning off the gas supply and bolting the front door when he goes out so that she should not do herself any injury or wander out into the street.'

The cumulative effect of the demands on the husband often produces frustration and anger, and when the husband's health also deteriorates, the strain cannot be sustained. Wives still attempt desperately to retain the remnants of their former roles. Social workers report, 'She goes crawling down the road with her husband to the shops'; or 'She manages to prop herself up against the sink and prepare a snack for them both', but sooner or later external help is sought.

The impact of ill health on the roles of spouses becomes clearer when one considers the way single people respond to hardships, not less severe than those affecting the married. A sixty-four-year-old bachelor, living on his own, suffers from heart trouble and acute diabetes, resulting in an amputated leg. He manages to confine his distress merely to the physical level. He does not preclude from his world the things he enjoys and cherishes, and those items which must be eliminated, like sporting activity, do not affect his overall self-evaluation. He does not feel accountable or responsible to other people, and this makes the problem of diminishing control over still significant elements of his life solely his affair. Indeed, as long as outside interference is avoided, his self-esteem is less likely to drop. This is well recognized by most single people, and the determination to retain independence at all costs, by not committing themselves to any group or individual, predominates in the management of their situation.

One problem shared by single people and couples alike, is that of undesirable accommodation. Even if the daily management of housekeeping is still within one's abilities, there are other aspects of living in a certain place which might create strain and anxiety leading to seeking suitable rehousing. A residence may become an unwanted burden as a result of either environmental difficulties or personal changes. Before pursuing these two contingencies any further, it is necessary to have some general idea of the housing conditions of the population in question. Table 1.10 presents some of the major features of types of accommodation occupied by the people attending the Centre according to sex and marital status.

The large proportion of people living on their own in houses, flats or bedsitters can give us a clue as to the widespread problems faced by them. These consist mainly of the need to deal with constant harassment by landlords or inversely with troublesome, recalcitrant, sometimes violent, tenants. In an area increasingly populated with various ethnic groups, there is a strong feeling of isolation stemming from the inability to communicate and to share the same values and interests. Fear of being attacked or mugged by wandering youths makes the finding of safe and Jewish accommodation one of the prime concerns of these people.

Even those who managed to rehouse themselves in a modern block of flats still confront the daunting possibility of facing an emergency when they are on their own, with no means of attracting attention to their plight, and no prospect of obtaining help. People who experienced blackouts, heart attacks, fits, etc. spread the recollection of their traumatic ordeal amongst elderly friends and impel them to look into the possibility of rehousing themselves yet again, in a safer residence.

As the conceived curtailment of independence in an old age home, and the slim chance of getting a place in one, discourage many people from considering this alternative, they look for flatlets controlled by a warden. This secures a reasonable degree of independence coupled with reliable safeguards in the event of an emergency. Hence, applications for flatlets occupy a great deal of the resources and concern of the social work done by the Jewish Welfare Board.

Emergencies and hostile environments are factors concerning

TABLE 1.10 *Type of accommodation (in percentages)*

Marital status	Houses		Flats		Flatlets		Bedsitters		Sharing		Unfixed address		Unknown	
Sex	m	f	m	f	m	f	m	f	m	f	m	f	m	f
Married	7.6	5.5	12	11.1	—	—	—	—	—	0.3	—	—	—	—
Widow/er	3.4	8.3	6.6	14	—	1.8	1.7	3.1	—	3.1	0.3	0.3	0.3	0.7
Unmarried	0.3	2.4	0.7	1	—	—	2	1.7	2	1.8	0.3	0.3	0.7	—
Separated and divorced	0.3	—	0.3	1.7	—	—	1.8	0.3	—	0.7	0.4	—	1.8	—
Total	11.6	16.2	19.6	27.8		1.8	5.5	5.1	2	5.9	1	—	2.8	0.7

Notes: (a) shared accommodation with children, parents or siblings;
(b) no fixed address — mainly sleeping rough;
(c) most of the flats are council accommodation and the majority of the houses are private property;
(d) people who were rehoused during the research period were tabled according to their longer residence.

the relationships between a person and other people. Yet, a person's accommodation also provides the setting of the relationship with himself. A house or a flat is not only shelter, but also a store of significant objects and memories. People who have lived together for more than a generation are not usually ready to encounter the new situation created when one of them passes away, or is taken into residential care. The strain of constantly confronting the missing person's traces, accompanied by the awareness that the relationships associated with these mementoes are never to be restored, may prove too much for some people to endure. The only escape is to leave these traces of the past behind, moving to another residence.

The non-material elements of the 'coping syndrome' are crucial, and a primary theme, the overriding problem of old people, is loneliness. Circumstances and personalities differ, but almost all the old people seeking help made this one of their main complaints. Isolation, desolation, loneliness and depression are common, often loosely used, descriptions for the vague and ill-defined predicament in which most elderly people find themselves. In fact loneliness and isolation are not synonymous, nor does the one necessarily imply the other. Townsend remarked (1973, p.189):

> To be socially isolated is to have few contacts with family and community. To be lonely is to have an unwelcome *feeling* of lack or loss of companionship. The one is objective the other is subjective ... the two do not coincide.

and: 'Some people living at the centre of a large family complained of loneliness and some who were living in extreme isolation repeated several times with vigour that they were never lonely' (ibid., p.195). There may indeed be a significant distinction between people who describe themselves as lonely and those who might be considered lonely by others, but not by themselves. In the Centre, single people who had led self-contained lives, and who had been spared the recent loss of someone close to them, were adamant that although their social life was restricted they never experienced loneliness.

My study suggests that most of the unmarried old people organized their immediate surroundings in such a way that only necessary daily items had been included. No objects associated with other people were found in their residences, and it appeared that for them the link between an object and its possessor had always been a direct one, no additional symbolic value stretching beyond its obvious instrumental importance. The range of significance of this kind of surrounding rests, therefore, within the boundaries of the surroundings themselves, which means that all the components involved in constructing it are controllable and manipulable.

Inversely, people who had lived for a long time – sometimes a life-time – with a person who had recently died, complained bitterly of loneliness regardless of the intensity of social contacts they had at the time. A widow who had visitors practically every hour of the day, married couples who had experienced a loss of a child, and a woman who had nursed her parents and sisters till they died, all described their present life in a house full of memories as intolerable. The list of possible examples is endless and corroborates the assumption that loneliness is fundamentally an acute feeling of deprivation accompanied by the realization that the balance between the desired and the controllable will never be redressed. The emotional strain involved in this imbalance is sometimes extremely difficult to sustain and a desperate reaction might occur. A woman whose husband died had developed a fervent belief that he was still alive, but had disappeared temporarily. She was very insistent in denying the social worker's suggestion that she was lonely. Another woman who had lost her mother firmly believed that she was convalescing in Israel and would return to her.

Nevertheless, these instances are fairly isolated cases. Most people who had suffered a loss of a close person expressed a strong sense of loneliness and were painfully aware of the irreversibility of their situation. Social workers and other concerned people try too often to fill in what seems to them the empty hours of loneliness with companionship and activity, but there is not a complete emptiness in loneliness. There is an unresolved strain, a feeling that although something important is missing, the other ingredients of the former situation are still in existence. This incongruity could not possibly be resolved by adding factors irrelevant and meaningless to the original shattered situation.

The following lines might demonstrate the extent of particularity involved in experiencing loneliness:

Retirement is near,
How will I spend my days without the company of you,

To me the cooking stove looks like some
Iron sculpture, seeing as I never had to cook, myself.

Remember, those summer evenings
Spent in Springfield Park together,
Gazing fondly at the children
Feeding ducks and geese.
O, how I appreciate you now you've gone
How long can my life go on.[6]

Loneliness, unsurprisingly, is regarded as a malady of old age, and it is indeed so, not only because of the high frequency of deaths amongst the elderly, but also due to the multiplexity of factors characterizing old age and liable to exacerbate loneliness. Retirement, ill health, a rejecting society, an alienating family and a non-supportive community, all play a role in accentuating the imbalance between one's world of relevant and meaningful things and people, and the ability to maintain viable, reciprocating relationships with it. It is impossible to gauge the extent or severity of something which is fundamentally a state of mind. However, there is enough ground to discern some differences both of degree and nature between lonely men and lonely women. Whereas the men are usually bitterly assertive in expressing the devastating effect of a recent loss in their life, the women express a more subdued, less clamorous appeal for help. The reason for this rests in the different relations between control and meaning attributable to men and women. Retirement, coupled by a death of a wife, indicates a major curtailment in a man's field of significance. A woman, on the other hand, merely faces retirement and the gradual relinquishment of her meaningful role as a housewife is not directly correlated with the absence of her husband. She can, therefore, still maintain a satisfactory relationship with her relevant environment without succumbing to the anomic reality a man might confront.

Perhaps the cardinal theme underpinning the 'coping' syndrome is concerned with the intense concentration on the day-to-day management of life in the face of a useless past and an uncertain future. People re-adjust their time-tables in a way which excludes making long term plans or leaning on past experiences. The apparent uselessness and irrelevance of past and future is not only a by-product of experiencing personal difficulties, but is also a product of encountering people's attitudes regarding the position

and the definition of the elderly in society. Such conceptions reinforce the overriding feeling of clinging to the present.

The end of involvement

The limbo state could be looked at from two different but complementary angles. One point of view is held by those who experience
it − in our case the aged − and the other is that shared by those
who produce and structure it, i.e. individuals and institutions associated directly or indirectly with old people. The way in which the
attitudes of the latter are conceived and construed by the old is
crucial in the construction of the limbo, in both the objective and
subjective sense.

This section will deal with some general conceptions of old
people as disseminated in different ways in the Centre and
absorbed and reacted to by its participants. Most of these images
relate to the position of the elderly and the disabled in society, and
have no special vernacular or denominational reference. As the
discussion is based strictly on the fieldwork data, it would be rather
presumptuous to attempt either a comprehensive analysis of the
place of the elderly in society or a sociological essay on the subject.
Instead I shall merely attempt to reflect on a number of values
concerning old age and prevailing amongst the people I studied.
Identification of these elements might allow us roughly to delineate
some of the cognitive boundaries of the limbo state and to inquire
further into the social factors defining it. Of the two interwoven
dimensions distilled in the constructions of any social definition −
the structural and the interactional − the first will be stressed here,
but the interactional perspective predominates in the book as a
whole. Here references to actual relationships and institutionalized
approaches to the elderly will be used simply to illustrate certain
values and general attitudes.

The following poem which was found amongst the possessions
of an old lady who had died in a geriatric hospital, and was distributed[7] and displayed in the Centre, provides a starting point as well
as an encapsulated panorama of the whole subject:

Crabbit Old Woman

What do you see nurses, what do you see,
    What are you thinking when you look at me?

A crabbit old woman, not very wise,
  Uncertain of habits with far-away eyes.
Who dribbles her food, and makes no reply
  When you say in a loud voice 'I do wish you'd try',
Who seems not to notice the things that you do,
  And forever is losing a stocking or shoe,
Who unresisting or not, lets you do as you will
  With bathing and feeding, the long day to fill.
Is that what you are thinking, is that what you see?
  Then open your eyes, you're not looking at me.
I'll tell you who I am as I sit here so still,
  As I move at your bidding, as I eat at your will.
I'm a small child of ten with a father and mother,
  Brothers and sisters who love one another.
A young girl at sixteen with wings at her feet,
  Dreaming that soon now a lover she'll meet.
A bride soon at twenty – my heart gives a leap.
  Remembering the vows that I promised to keep.
At twenty-five now I have young of my own,
  Who need me to build a secure happy home.
A woman of thirty may now grow fast,
  Bound to each other with ties that should last.
At forty my young now will soon be gone
  But my man stays beside me to see I don't mourn.
At fifty once more babies play round my knee.
  Again we know children, my loved one and me.

Dark days are upon me, my husband is dead.
  I look at the future, I shudder with dread.
For my young are all busy rearing young of their own
  And I think of the years and the love I have known.
I'm an old woman now and nature is cruel,
  'tis her jest to make old age look like a fool.
The body it crumbles, grace and vigour depart.
  And now there's stone where I once had a heart.
But inside this old carcase a young girl still dwells,
  And now and again my battered heart swells,
I remember the jobs, I remember the pain,
  And I'm loving and living life over again.
I think of the years all too few – gone so fast,

And accept the stark fact that nothing can last.
So open your eyes nurses, open and see,
Not a crabbit old woman, look closer — see *me*.

Needless to say that these lines contain more than could be included
in a limited sociological discussion. Nevertheless, certain themes
should be pointed out. The last span of the woman's life cycle is
associated with a poignant incongruity between her self-conception
and the way she is looked upon by the people who look after her.
This unbridgeable gap is created not only because of obvious difficulties in communicating with other people, but is mainly due to a
widespread conception of old people as being bundles of needs and
demands, mere non-reciprocating recipients.

A film produced by the Jewish Welfare Board and shown at the
Centre blatantly presented this attitude. A young man appeared on
the screen and in crude and harsh terms described old people as a
non-contributing, ever-consuming part of society. This feeling of
being an unwanted burden on society is well recognized by participants; as one of them put it, 'the only crime I have committed is
growing old'. The subject of redundancy is often broached in
discussion groups and other Centre encounters and is invariably
referred to in terms of bitter realization and acceptance of the
socially imposed inferiority.

The receiving status of old people poses no problem to the
conveyors of social provisions, i.e. social workers and the like. On
the contrary, relating to a special need is not as complicated and
frustrating as dealing with a whole personality. Nevertheless awareness of this situation preoccupies many social workers and some of
them have developed an apologetic response, whereby the attitude
of viewing old people merely in the light of their material needs is
projected onto the clients, who are conceived as highly engrossed
with their immediate physical and financial conditions.

The 'Age Concern' plea[8] is that we should not consider old
people 'a race apart'. The reduction of the aged to their physical
limitations is one of the commonest determinants of this segregation, and members of the medical profession, being in frequent
contact with the elderly, are amongst the principal agents who
make the social evaluation apparent. Medical advice to elderly
patients, implying their uselessness and predestined deterioration,
makes the awareness of physical reduction almost inevitable.

Doctors' authoritative and decisive statements such as, 'you are good only for dominoes and draughts' and 'there are no jobs for a man in your condition', forestall any attempt by the patient to define his general situation differently, particularly since the medical opinion usually contains some directives about how to live out one's life, given one's physical state.

Reducing the social image of old people to basic physical and material necessities manifests itself in endless encounters involving the elderly. Forced retirement, redundancy, produces a feeling of rejection. Attempts to resume a working life often provoke curt rebuffs, like 'don't bother us any more, you are not fit enough for any job'. These clinch the realization that this important, almost taken-for-granted aspect of life, is beyond recovery. The effect of an abrupt discontinuation of a working relationship was succinctly expressed by a participant in a discussion group on retirement: 'the world was not my world'.

The reluctant disengagement from that old world is socially accomplished by categorizing the redundant under certain collective labels implying a sharp distinction from other sectors of society and awarding a definite legal and normative status to the people included. Thus allocation to the 'Senior Citizens' 'Old Folk' 'OAP.' categories, although entailing some indisputable material benefits and rights, contains an unmistakable insinuation that this marks the end of any significant involvement and participation in making decisions affecting their own life.

Granting special concessions and privileges to old people does not obliterate their presence and the constant attention they need foils any attempt to disentangle them completely from the 'contributing' sectors of society. This presents a problem as to what attitudes and patterns of behaviour should be adopted in the course of encounters and dealings involving old people. There are no specifically defined roles established on professional, economic or political grounds to which one can refer whilst communicating with the elderly. Therefore, any message containing more than official notification of regulations based on statutory legislation requires an accepted code, different from that used in addressing better socially defined people.

One way of relating to old people is by obliterating their life history and social identity, and reducing them to their physical and mental disabilities. Thus applicants to the old age homes of the

Jewish Welfare Board are classified strictly according to these criteria. Well-defined yardsticks are used to assess the suitability of a client for a specific home. All the components of this assessment are meant to predict the applicant's response to the imposed environmental conditions to which he might be subjected. The list of factors taken into account in considering an application includes none even remotely germane to the client's ability to contribute to the home, nor do they concern attributes in areas of no concern to the staff. The factors considered relevant are: Physical: mobility, dressing, feeding, continence, sleep; Mental: orientation, communication, co-operation, restlessness and mood. Irrespective of the way the assessment is implemented, the list consistently eliminates the old person's other social qualities and idiosyncrasies.

Regimenting old people in institutions may alleviate the problem of daily dealings caused by their presence amongst the non-aged, but it does not mitigate the need to find a satisfactory way of interacting with them whilst avoiding the ambiguity engrained in their socially undefined position.

One mechanism, marked in the life of the Centre, but undoubtedly prevailing outside it, is provided by the frequently drawn analogy between old people and children. The sociological resemblance although too intriguing to be overlooked, is beyond the scope of this discussion. Nevertheless, some of the patterns adopted by members of staff and outsiders to relate to participants were guided by the paradigm of the relationship with children. Thus, the first suggestion to boost activities amongst participants made by a new administrator introduced to the Centre was to arrange documentary and Walt Disney film shows 'like they used to do in my old school'. The bingo organized by outside volunteers was opened by the well-known phrase used to children 'Are you sitting comfortably? Then we'll begin'. On another occasion – a Sunday tea arranged by outsiders – small gifts in birthday-like packets were distributed amongst those attending. A member of staff refused to join the participants in an outing to a pantomime claiming that that sort of show was only for children. An abortive attempt was made to organize an open day at the Centre to display the participants' work and activities on the implicit model of similar occasions in schools.

Social workers' reports on elderly clients are rife with remarks and attitudes associating old people with children. Comments such as 'a sweet old lady', 'inadequate person', 'well-adapted', 'positive personality', 'most uncomplaining old lady', etc. present personality assessments based on the client's contrary or obliging response to the social worker's conception of the appropriate treatment for him.

However, two major discrepancies exist between the social position of children and that of the aged. The first is that children have no past experience of involvement and power to which they can compare their present deprived situation. The old, however, have both the experience and awareness with which to confront and judge their present circumstances. This awareness is accompanied by the realization that it is an irrevocable situation, which causes explicit feelings of frustration, inferiority, shame and indignity.

The second incongruity in the analogy involves another aspect of society's attitude towards the two categories. Whilst children, being in a transitional stage of their life, are expected and encouraged to show constant progress and eventually to join the ranks of their instructors, no such process of socialization is designed or even contemplated for the elderly. On the contrary, their social and personal state is regarded as a permanent one with only one direction of change – physical and mental deterioration. Hence, as far as the non-aged are concerned, the elderly, sustained by the provisions of the welfare services, are in a stage of inert stagnation, euphemistically described as 'peace and tranquillity'.

To warrant this attitude and maybe also to gain some 'moral absolution'[9] a few social mechanisms have been developed. Two of them are particularly relevant to our discussion. The first is the intensive effort spent on promoting recreational activities amongst the aged. Resources are directed to provide various facilities to enable elderly people to get together and 'pass their time' in a way which has no effect on their involvement with other parts of society. The assertion that 'clubs and social centres exist for *all* old people to increase social contact and to give scope and facilities for new pursuits in retirement'[10] contains a number of elements fundamental to the origins of this social sequestration.

There is the indiscriminate approach to '*all* old people'. There is also the assumption that elderly people seek social contact for its own sake and participate in occupational therapy, discussion groups and the like first and foremost for the companionship they may offer. The idea of sheer friendship has been reiterated on numerous occasions and has been professed by staff and members alike to be the main factor attracting new participants to the Centre. This last premise is a predominant one in moulding patterns of treating old people, and is probably the rudimentary motivation upon which day care for the elderly is devised; this is to assume that members would attend these establishments for the simple pleasure of meeting other people, regardless of other benefits which might be gained by such encounters, and with no other purpose in mind.

The following quotation taken from a Jewish Welfare Board fund-raising advertisement could illuminate this last point:[11]

HELP GIVE THE ONE MEDICINE A DOCTOR CAN'T
The invaluable prescription of human company which is provided at a JWB Day Centre.
Basically this is a place for old folk to spend the day.
But look a bit deeper, and you'll find all these benefits.
At lunchtime a Day Centre gives many pensioners their only hot meal of the day.
And provides the companionship − without which many old people living alone die mentally, years before their time.
And because an elderly relative can be cared for at a Day Centre, a housewife might well be free to take a much-needed job.
In all these ways − and more − a JWB Day Centre acts as a safety valve.
It relieves a situation which we know can lead to so many problems − medical and financial.
This is really practical valuable work … .

The juxtaposition between the two explicit functions a day centre is meant to fulfil − that of providing companionship and that of a social 'safety valve' − is too salient to be coincidental. As it is regarded as rather inappropriate to define old age homes and day care establishments for the purpose they really serve, i.e. disposal units for non-productive, socially isolated people, the imputed striving for companionship has been used to legitimize their existence, and to satisfy the need for self-righteousness and clear conscience. Indeed, caring for the elderly is a product of a certain value system interwoven with a changing social structure, but it is quite evident that this care is as beneficial to the 'do gooders' as to the recipients.

Establishing social 'safety valves' is only one justification for the socially imposed state of stagnation. The second, although not as widely accepted as the first one, enables its advocates to take a very passive noncommittal line in their dealings with the elderly. This is the premise that part of the process of getting old is an increased state of self-satisfaction and intrinsic contentment. Social workers have commented on some of their clients that, despite their psychological anguish and social deprivation, they are fundamentally happy. A talk given at the Centre followed by a short film showed a hostel for the disabled whose residents were capable of doing and making anything regardless of their handicap. The general picture was of a happy contented community able to enjoy life to the full. Another film show, whilst designed to make old people aware of traffic regulations, featured the contrast between the aftermath of an accident and the happy tranquil life the victim had led previously. The theme was there is too much happiness and fulfilment at stake in later life to put it at risk in a preventable calamity.

A song written by a member of another day centre, sung with much relish and solidarity by our participants, counts the many 'special' attributes of that day centre:

> Special supervisors ... Special welfare coaches with special fitted rails. A special place for wheelchairs and special lifted rails. There are special expert drivers and special escorts too and if you need some special help they know just what to do ... a special ramp especially for chairs. There are always special helpers to move the chairs around. A special lift for everyone who can't get up the stairs ... A very special dining room and special dinners too, and if you're on a diet these are specially for you. A special canteen worker will bring a special sweet, and if you're too handicapped she'll even cut your meat.

and so on and so forth.[12] The conclusion is 'so come along and join us, we are quite a happy throng. Come and have some fun with us ...'. This assertion is reiterated in the refrain:

> We are all happy at the Centre,
> We are all happy at the Centre,
> We are all happy at the Centre and so say all of us.

The evident link between the 'special' sheltered environment the Centre provides and the happiness its participants claim to enjoy might give us a clue as to the nature of that happiness.

Old people being included in a well-protected, adequately provided for social category, are regarded as self-sufficient individuals
who need care and attention, but are exempted from any further
responsibility and commitment. They are thought of as people
who, unlike most members of society, have very little control over
their surroundings and nothing to which to aspire. They disengage
themselves from the competitive dynamic scene of conflicts, confrontations and discontent and, therefore, should consider themselves satisfied, with no cause for real unhappiness stemming from
competition for status and power.

This view has been strongly seconded by participants whose lives
have been constituted very much along this line of no responsibility, no aspirations and hopes and no obligations. Quite a number
of them confessed their full satisfaction and their willingness to
remain in that state despite the awareness that by doing so they
inevitably excluded themselves from a whole range of social involvements and previous relationships.

Smith-Blau (1973, p. 152) cynically points out that 'many people
"gracefully" accept being "farmed out to pasture" for the remaining fifteen or twenty years of their "one and only life cycle". They
"accept" their fate in the existing social order. When asked they
purport to be "satisfied" with life ... . They are told after all that
disengagement is normal and inevitable with ageing.' Indeed, the
controversy over 'Disengagement Theory' (Cumming and Henry,
1961), acclaimed by Parsons and fervently disputed by others, con-
firms that this view of old people as a happy, uncomplaining
minority dominates some conceptions of the elderly in our society,
and sustains people who are engaged in the sphere of the aged.

Yet with due respect to the attitudes expressed by the elderly and
the arduous scientific effort spent in processing and theorizing
about them, there is no conclusive evidence as to the nature of the
happiness old people are alleged to enjoy and, therefore, the relevant data and discussions should be taken as another facet of the
social tenet that old pople are satisfied with their stagnant position.
And as Smith-Blau (1973, pp. 152-3) indicates: 'it can so easily be
used as a rationale by the non-old, who constitute the "normals" in
society, to avoid confrontation and dealing with the issue of old
people's marginality and rolelessness.'

The constitution of the happy social deadlock of the elderly is based upon one major set of rules — the elimination and obliteration of any element associated with progress, competition, tension and productivity. Any infraction of these rules by introducing one of these ingredients into the limbo state is regarded as an usurpation of the rights of the non-old, and is sanctioned accordingly.

Those elements provided and controlled by society (such as jobs, accommodation, status symbols) present no specific problem, as they are all monitored and controlled by the non-aged. However, there are some other aspects of life which are considered to be the sole privilege of the non-old, but might be abutted upon by the old and thus could shatter the whole flimsy borderline created by the non-old to differentiate themselves from the aged.

The most commonly cited example of this danger is the attitude towards sexual activities amongst the elderly. People who are in charge of the daily handling of old people frequently come across cases of clients who continue or resume sexual interest. Invariably the reaction is surprise sometimes mixed with shock and disgust. Some of them consider indulgence a disruptive element in institutional life, and treat it as a disturbance which should be eradicated. A client who had been found by a social worker sitting in his room surrounded by pin-ups was referred to as 'a dirty old man', and female colleagues were advised not to take up his case. A matron who found a resident masturbating called upon the head-office staff to assist her in tackling the 'problem' and to prevent other residents from following that man's example.

The social enclave for the elderly is confined and maintained by the translation of attitudes and approaches into modes and patterns of behaviour and treatment, applied to the aged within the overriding framework supplied by the welfare state. It is far beyond the scope of this discussion to explore the factors involved in the historical development of modern social policies. However, some considerations of the repercussions of these policies are highly pertinent to the understanding of the social position of the elderly at present and particularly concern those of them — like the Centre participants — who, due to their generally inadequate private means, are forced to take full advantage of such provisions.

State benefits coupled with local authorities' domiciliary and residential services permeate all aspects of life. A brief list of available provisions show that there is hardly an area of material needs which is not covered by them. Ranging from contributory pensions, non-contributory benefits, allowances and grants to 'meals on wheels', visiting district nurse, holidays and clubs, these provisions encircle the elderly with safeguards against most of the shortages entailed by the process of ageing in our society.

The accessibility of these resources depends on adequate information, some personal initiative, or the concern of other people, plus the ability to overcome the barrier of shame and indignity involved in applying for some of these services. Most of these factors are within the old person's control and it is up to him to decide whether, or not, to take advantage of the whole gamut. This produces a major change in a person's concept of his relationship with his environment. There is no longer reciprocity, but a fixed receipt with no return.

This form of one-sided dependency impregnates other spheres of relationships in which the elderly are involved, especially that of the old person with his offspring. The responsibility for the care of the aged has been diverted from children to the state regardless of the will and means of the former, and hence a long-standing obligation on the part of children to provide for their ageing parents has become virtually devoid of all substantial content. The temptation to utilize the provisions offered by the state is too tantalizing to be ignored by both parents and children and the inevitable result is that, although concern and interest might still be shown by children, there is no longer a need for them to include the elderly in their daily life. Thus, two separate, self-contained entities are created out of what used to be an interwoven world.

This is a further step in the process of detachment and segregation. As there is no reciprocity between the aged and their providers, it is often unrecognized by the latter that the static change-resisting nature imputed by them to the elderly is more of a reflection of their own attitudes and policies than a true picture of reality. In fact, old people are in the course of a most dynamic changeable phase of life and as they perceive and accept the view that they are immutable, an intriguing contradiction is created between the self-conception of the elderly and the actual situation they are in. This is relevant to the way in which old people respond to social isolation coupled with unarrested deterioration.

Choice

The course of action differs in form, intensity and repercussions. It might be designed to combat one isolated difficulty, like applying for home-help services to facilitate housework, or it might encapsulate all aspects of life, such as admission into an old age home. The options open to people and the factors involved in choosing between them are the subject of the following section.

There is a whole range of potential determinants affecting a decision. The precipitating factor is, however, an awareness that the problem exists, and that it is beyond one's powers to carry on leading the sort of life one used to live. A change is imperative. A few people are struck by this awareness after a dramatic, unexpected mishap, such as a death of a close person, or an abrupt illness, but in most instances people just face a gradual, consistent deterioration. However, some recurrent characteristics could be roughly outlined as cues in the transformation leading to seeking help.

The ominous feeling of loneliness and depression described earlier is usually substituted and followed by a state which social workers as well as participants tend to call 'self-pity'. It is recognized that feeling sorry for oneself is a negative, shameful and destructive state of mind, making a transition between the realistic acceptance of limitations and abilities and a paralysing, total submission to loneliness and depression. This signals the rudimentary realization that some improvement could and should be sought.

A man who lost his wife described the change in his self-conception as a transformation from an overall incapacity to perform any function usually fulfilled by his late wife, to attempting to take her place in looking after himself by cooking, doing the daily household chores, etc. 'I realized that my depression was mostly self-pity and I could take care of myself if I wanted to.'

In the eyes of social workers self-pity is unwarranted. The client could, if he so wished, help himself more than he appeared to do:

'Very lonely and depressed and full of self-pity – mourning problem. After having lived an active business life feels useless and unwanted. Has not made much of an adjustment to life at home and cannot cope with having nothing to do. Feels a burden on her family. Placing obstructions in the way of helping herself e.g. by refusing convalescence holidays offered on several occasions.'

The association in the report between self-pity and rejecting convalescence is essential to the understanding of the awareness of self-pity as the initial realization that a meaningful long term solution is to be pursued instead of an ephemeral non-committal response. This rejection of temporary measures is significantly common amongst people who are in pursuit of ways and means to tackle their difficulties in a more decisive manner than that of short term reprieves.

The feeling of being an unwanted burden on other people marks the emergence of another stage in the building up of awareness, that is a profound poignant disappointment with almost all people and institutions with which the affected person has had some contact. It ranges from alienated families and disobliging friends and neighbours to inattentive doctors and uninterested community establishments. This is a stage of shattered expectations and increased isolation. People begin to put to the test other people's commitments and loyalties and the disappointing result is often a cause for a further withdrawal from former engagements and ties.

The major change perhaps is the new perspective gained by the elderly on their exchange relationships with their environment. Undoubtedly, rejection and desertion by family is the most devastating and bitter disappointment of all. It is a widely expressed opinion amongst the Centre participants that children in the 'old times', namely themselves, were brought into the world to provide their parents with some security for the future. So much so that some parents deliberately chose different trades for their offspring in order that unemployment and economic recession would not have the same affect on all the children, so that at least one of them would be sufficiently comfortably-off to support his parents. The unresponsive attitude of their own children puts in grave doubt the balance of give and take between them; and people start questioning the whole nature of the relationship.

Thus as a past relationship carries no obligation for the present, the whole basis of their family concept is at stake. The same applies to friends and neighbours. An inevitable review of these relationships occurs when, while facing a crisis situation like severe illness or bereavement, neither help nor concern is rendered by friends and neighbours. A complete disregard shown by synagogue authorities and other denominational organizations precipitate and seal the new realization that one is living in an estranged non-supportive environment and, therefore, should be as self-reliant as possible.

This leads to a subsequent stage in the process of awareness, increasing disenchantment giving way to an explicit expression of acrimony and cynicism. Life-long ties are seen in a new, unfavourable light and the awkward task of maintaining them seems to be meaningless. This produces a deliberate attempt to disentangle oneself from no longer desirable involvements; parents cease to telephone their children who do not visit them. Some refrain from going to synagogues even on major festivals. Friends and neighbours are practically written-off.

This disengagement is also associated with a newly adopted attitude of mistrust and suspicion towards all agents of the helping profession. As formerly accepted criteria of social esteem and self-evaluation are discredited the shame normally attached to dependency on social services, especially to those offered by the Jewish Welfare Board, diminishes. The removal of this barrier is essential to the initiation of any application for assistance.

Analytically this mode of transformation from depression to realization could be seen also as a process through which a person divorces his own conception of self from that attributed to him by his social environment. As reflections on past experience elicit no adequate response to present stresses and changes, the individual develops a self-evaluation which, almost paradoxically, corresponds with prevailing social conceptions of the elderly as roleless people. An unavoidable disjunction occurs between what Mead (1939) called 'me' and the 'I', i.e. between the objective, socially formed aspect of self, and the subjective, ingrained facet of personality.

This abstraction of the general, but by no means unitary formation of awareness is exemplified in the following two examples of pre-Centre situations:

John was an unmarried man of seventy with no family, living on his own. He enjoyed good health, an active social life – 'I had thousands of friends' – a thriving business, and a car. Of his own accord he decided to sell the business and to retire to a peaceful, comfortable life.

At the beginning he used to fill his time with social activities and reading, but gradually he found himself increasingly bored and uninterested. He lost his appetite. An attempt to have a meal in a well-known Jewish restaurant ended with his expulsion on the grounds that his overt aversion to the food would put off other customers. Severe emaciation accompanied by constipation and painful urinating difficulties weakened John to the extent of fainting, and yet his doctor found nothing physically wrong with him.

One evening, suffering from excruciating pain and general frailty, he tried to get in to a hospital. He crawled into the street dressed in his pyjamas and reached his car on all fours. Passersby avoided him and no help was offered. Motorists hooted at him and his dangerous driving eventually drew the attention of a policeman who stopped him for a breathalser test. When he arrived at the hospital he was told that he would need surgical interference and consequently he would remain incontinent. At that stage John decided that his life was not worth living and asked the doctor for euthanasia. The reaction was a laughing dismissal.

He was operated upon and unexpectedly the outcome was not as anticipated, and his biological functions were restored to normal. John made up his mind to rebuild his life, accepting that he should not expect any concern or help from other people. As John expressed it, 'I have been barred from the restaurant, the policeman didn't believe that I wasn't a drunk, and in the hospital I was treated like a bit of rubbish.'

Social workers who had seen to John disputed his version of these events, but John's presentation of his plight is relevant, whatever the objective facts. Whilst reflecting on the building up of his pre-Centre state, he chose to pick up certain points which correspond with other participants' views of their pre-Centre conditions.

Unlike John, who retired of his own volition and was in control of events until his illness, Jack was subject to a series of blows. He was involved in a road accident which crippled him and forced him to retire from his job as a taxi-driver. His wife fell ill, and was bedridden for two years, requiring constant care and nursing from her husband. In addition to all this, Jack was afflicted by a severe heart condition. The death of his wife left him extremely depressed and as a result he was hospitalized in a mental ward. Electro-Convulsive Treatment was applied to him several times.

In Jack's terms he was 'no more a human being but a vegetable, I could not call myself alive, I didn't care about anything'. Having been discharged from hospital he had spent his days in complete seclusion at his flat in a council 'tower block' where he did not see a soul for days.

Again, verification of the story would seem impertinent to the way Jack conceives his pre-Centre existence. These two men had reached the stage of awareness of their situation which led to action to improve it by entering the Centre, through a contact with a social worker established for them by the hospital. Other people had found their way to the Centre via other channels, like local authorities, previous connections with the Jewish Welfare Board, indirect referrals made by family and neighbours, etc.

The Centre is by no means the first and only venture people make as a result of their newly gained awareness of their situation. There are alternative and complementary reactions, some of them mutually exclusive, others not. Before examining the variety of possibilities, let us go through some of the main factors involved in making the decision to try one or more of them and to overlook others.

Awareness may be seen as the realization that the gap between the things one can control and those which are still relevant and meaningful to one's life, but uncontrollable, is irretrievable. The action taken is usually an attempt to change the relationship between field of relevance and level of control, so that the strain exerted by the incompatibility will be diminished. Two interlinked sets of factors determine the nature of the measures finally taken.

The first include factors within one's personal control. Although the specific type of problems one confronts is itself a fundamental determinant, the attitude adopted towards them plays an important role in the making of the decision. An amputation as a result of severe diabetes might lead either to a strong determination not to let the disease overshadow one's life, and to limit its impact to the necessary treatments and technical adjustments, or to a complete withdrawal to a world centred around the illness and governed by a constant engrossment with its physical, social and mental implications.

A person's reaction to such an affliction is necessarily dependent on the means at his disposal. Money can be used to combat the particular hardships. If limited mobility necessitates some help around the house, one can either hire a daily, or apply for a 'home-help' from local authorities. The former solution, which is obviously the more expensive, would involve limited social implications whereas the latter would probably entail some change in one's self-evaluation. However, few of the people in question have adequate financial means, and private means can be left out of account in the range of options open.

Most of the elderly in the area suffer from more than one problem which makes options more complicated, and leads to a search for a comprehensive 'solution'. Only in a few cases are people able and willing to arrive at such major decisions (such as entering an old age home) on their own initiative. Thus relationships with other people and institutions become relevant.

The intricate relationship with the family dominates almost any major decision, particularly the possibility of admission to a residential institution. Pressure is often exerted by children both on social workers and on the parent, and the welfare of the elderly applicant is only one of the factors considered. The prospect of getting hold of property, especially the house owned by the parents, is often a consideration, as is the fear that the parent might become a burden on the family.

Other social agents whose involvement with the old impinges on the choice of action are members of the helping professions. Doctors, hospital social workers, health inspectors, home-helps, community workers, etc. give advice and make referrals to other agencies. Their actual compulsory power is rather limited, but in the absence of other support and concern their clients become highly dependent on their visits and connections and, therefore, are inclined to follow their guidance.

These agents act also as the main source of information about the possible short and long term solutions, the existence and availability of benefits and the ways to go about claiming them. Luncheon clubs, workshops for the elderly, library home services and the other day care facilities all come to the knowledge of the people for whom they are designed through contact with members of this category. The selection of resources depends on the other factors I have mentioned, and there is always room for an individual, non-institutional course of action in coping with the widening gulf between relevance and control.

One sort of initiative, though uncommon, is worth looking into since it demonstrates the reluctance to accept the inexorable existence of the gap and to become reconciled to it. It applies mostly to people who were self-employed and did not have to face forced retirement. Some of them try to resume working, either in their own business or in a workshop for the elderly. A return to self-employment usually yields inadequate income, and adversely affects their health. Sheltered workshops provide a rather limited range of activity requiring no initiative, offer little financial and social incentive, and involve a strong element of self-degradation.

Avoidance of confronting the gap is another common reaction. Some people try to forestall any situation which might expose them to the poignant incongruity. Thus, they spend most of the day outside the home, not cooking and washing there but rather using the available substitutes, like luncheon clubs, public baths and launderettes. The home, therefore, is gradually reduced to fulfilling the function merely of a roof over the head, and thereby the risk of encountering relics and memories from a conceived harmonious, but irretrievable past is reduced.

A conceivable response to the imbalance between diminishing ability and an existing world of importance would be to rationalize the gap by means of some sort of ideology. This is rare. The stage of awareness amongst these people does not include a strong conceptual, explanatory element. Obviously one readily available system of ideas and symbols which might be used to bridge the gap, is religion. However, people in the Centre were critical of the Jewish religious establishment, and disenchanted with synagogues. Any resort to religious practice or thinking was looked upon in a most unfavourable light. (See 'alternative realities', below.) No more than a handful of people have adopted the attitude that their present plight is God's will, which should be accepted and respected. Such people also express their confidence that the imbalance will be redressed at another time in another world. One might say then that for them there is some obscure meaning to their hardship and, since that future is thought to include an after-life, the experience of time is not as aimless as other peoples'.

Restoration of a working life, avoidance of the home, and rationalization are the less common ways of facing up to the new awareness. Most of the other reactions are aimed at a direct intervention to alter the field of relevance, the range of control, or both. The search for new relations can take various forms. The least tried is a fundamental alteration of values and beliefs, i.e. a change of orientation from no longer controllable relevant objects to those likely to be responsive and achieved. Concentrating on 'petty things', going into minute 'unimportant details', focusing attention on marginal points − all regarded as sure signs of 'senility' and 'mental deterioration' − could be seen as a part of the attempt to change relevance in order to achieve some compatibility with control. Obviously this can succeed only when supported by social encounters with other people sharing the same desire to reconstruct their world of relevance. This might be managed through participation in clubs, and establishing social contacts with other elderly people, but individual adjustments can modify the relation between control and relevance.

There is always the retreatist reaction widely discussed in relevant literature and generally known as 'withdrawal' or 'second childhood', 'wandering off', etc. This is the belief that old people are predisposed to sink into a constant state of reminiscing, oblivious to the world and divorced from awareness of causation. As depicted by Smith-Blau (1973, p. 155) 'A retreatist frequently "daydreams of the past", enjoys "just sitting and thinking about things" and is "absent minded". He is the escapist *par excellence*.' Irrespective of biological processes involved in the creation of this state, the fact that many of these 'daydreamers' have 'awakened' at the Centre by clinging to the present, as will be described further on, implies that it is fundamentally a response to a social situation, a response aimed at obliterating completely the field of control whilst becoming excessively and solely engrossed with an expanded, meaningful field of relevance.

Retreatism is often the precursor of an application for a place in an old age home. This may be made either by the family, supported or challenged by the social worker, or by the elderly person himself. An outside initiative is basically a matter of exerting pressure on the candidate in an attempt to put him away for reasons of convenience to the family, whereas a personal application indicates a move to make the state of retreat a permanent, sheltered one.

The image of residential institutions for the elderly as places of inertia and decadence (Townsend, 1964) or 'Tombs for the Living' (Henry, 1972, p. 321) is widespread amongst social workers, who often go out of their way to dissuade clients from entering such an establishment. Their main argument is the inevitable complete loss of autonomy and independence built into the institutional regime. Nevertheless, very few clients have changed their mind as a result of such arguments. The reason is probably that residential care would not necessarily signify a curtailment of independence, but rather a continuation of an exciting condition of decreasing control. Entering an old age home means no more deterioration, but rather a secure, predictable environment, within which an undisturbed retreat is feasible. In fact, in many cases applicants look forward to the change which means to them a carefree life with no family harassment, or frustrated attempts to struggle with an increasingly harsh daily routine.

However, faced with progressive inability to cope, the commonest reaction is to find a new environment in which certain difficulties are eliminated without total relinquishment of autonomy and independence. This middle-range solution is offered by warden-controlled 'flatlets'. Here residents are allowed to lead fully independent lives whilst some services, advice and, mainly, security in case of an emergency, are provided by the warden. Some people, however, adopt a cynical approach to the world whilst leading non-committal, almost nomadic lives, moving aimlessly from one Salvation Army hostel to another or around parks and tube stations. For some of these people the idea of being accommodated under any form of supervision is distasteful.

When people come to the Centre they have experience of some of these reactions and the new experiment is looked upon with much suspicion and a tinge of cynicism. They know vaguely that it might help them to overcome loneliness, to get a cheap hot meal, and that it provides opportunities for small-talk and craft work. But does the reality in the Centre offer more than that? What are the relations between the problems characterizing the pre-Centre situation and the Centre world?

With the exception of religion and one or two eccentric individual enterprises,[13] all the reactions discussed offer merely temporary and partial relief to the strain and predicaments embedded in the pre-Centre situation. The Centre is an arena for another range of responses, of quite a different nature, and as this new setting is cognate with the essence of the limbo state, it is appropriate to make a precis of the main features underpinning the pre-Centre situation.

The crux is the incongruity between the static role imputed to and imposed on the elderly by their social environment, and the constant experience of change of disintegration and deterioration. Were it not for this contradiction, elderly people, like some other underprivileged minorities,[14] would probably have complied with their unfavourable static position. As it is, incompatibility between social definition and reality engenders amongst the aged awareness, examination and defiance.

The widening gap between relevance and control is one aspect of that incongruity. In the absence of socially formulated alternative realities, the dearth of means of interacting with one's significant environment becomes critical. Social attitudes and constraints forestall any real prospect of arresting deterioration, and the 'solutions' offered are simply a reflection of its origins: i.e. avoidance, reducing the individual to his limitations and confining him to a social cul-de-sac. The elderly, therefore, are confronted with two conflicting dimensions of time. Their position in society consists of static elements whereas the unavoidable process of disintegration changes conditions and abilities. The individual facing the irreconcilable contradiction is presented with a fundamental twofold existential problem concerning both his self-conception and his experience of time. The first relates to the disengagement between the aged and the non-aged, whilst the second involves further aspects of this process such as its implication for one's perspectives on one's life history, present ties and affiliations, and future potential.

There is one added time dimension which has not yet been dealt with, but should be noted here. There is little doubt that the proximity of impending death impinges heavily upon the elderly person's conception of time. Recurrent losses of spouses and friends, daily confrontations with hospitals, worsening ill health and the certainty of constant deterioration, are all interlinked contributions to the realization that life is an accelerated sequence of uncontrollable changes heading towards an inevitable end. Disenchantment and awareness rob this realization of any acceptable meaning.

This time factor in the life of the elderly has been scantily discussed in the relevant sociological and psychological literature.[15] Role approaches and adjustment theories offer a marginal insight into the subject, and recent attempts (Kimmel, 1974) to use concepts borrowed from symbolic interaction relate mainly to the interrelations between the components of self, almost excluding the germane social aspects. None the less, the dimension of time has been dealt with to some extent as part of discussions on the structure of the life cycle. Erikson (1959, p. 98) whilst discussing the negative resolution of the final stage of life – identity diffusions – writes, 'Despair expresses the feeling that the time is short, too short for the attempt to start another life, and to try out an alternative road to integrity.' Neugarten (1968) by suggesting the concept of the 'social clock' as a regulator and monitor of change and progress in the individual's life cycle, implies in fact that as far as the elderly are concerned that 'clock' is non-existent for there are no expectations or sanctions relating to their management of time.[16]

The lack of social time interlinked with the other ramifications of disintegration and diminishing control affect the way in which participants constitute their social world in the Centre. This world will be viewed through the prism of the participants' time universe and hence will be considered as a reaction to their temporal dilemma. None the less, I would not argue that the Centre adjustment is inevitable or necessary. The process of awareness discussed earlier, although perhaps indicating a cognitive link between the predicament of the limbo state and the course of action taken to resolve it, is by no means the sole determinant of the type and content of response. The particular pattern of behaviour and attitudes developed in the Centre, as will be described in the following sections, emerges both from pre-Centre situations and from the nature of the Centre environment.

2 The setting

The ways in which people in the Centre encounter the limbo state follow from the basic nature of the pre-Centre situation, and the social arena created by the Centre.

The Centre as a sociological phenomenon is a hybrid, formed by the participants' behaviour and a combination of environmental circumstances. These circumstances include: the conception of social work and of its recipients current in the Centre; the relationships within the staff; the resources and opportunities open to participants; and the relationship between the Centre and the outside world. All these dimensions are relevant in the daily running of the Centre. A brief profile of the mode of participation, the premises, the facilities, the routine and the history of the Centre will reveal the factors responsible for its transformation from a temporary sanctuary for the lonely and the poor into a vital core around which their total lives revolve.

The Centre

Applications to the Centre are made through various channels and handled by members of the Jewish Welfare Board's team of social workers operating in the Marlsden area. Nevertheless, a large number of participants approach the Centre directly simply by entering the premises and mingling with its members, and any attempt to describe the avenues through which people are introduced would be incomplete without some consideration of the haphazard factor involved in admission to the Centre.

The data in Table 2.1 on referrals to the Centre relates only to 290 participants out of the approximately 350 who attend it every week. It would be reasonable to assume that the remaining 60 have had very little contact, or none at all, with the staff. Most of them are irregular members visiting the Centre every now and again, or

TABLE 2.1 *Referrals to the Centre according to sex and marital status (in percentages)*

Marital status	Way of referring to the Centre												
	A		B		C		D		E		F		G	
	m	f	m	f	m	f	m	f	m	f	m	f	m	f
Married	0.6	0.6	—	0.9	4.6	4.7	2.9	1.0	4.0	6.0	2.1	2.1	—	—
Widows and widowers	—	3.2	6.0	5.6	3.1	6.0	1.0	0.5	9.0	11.0	1.1	3.2	—	0.7
Unmarried	—	—	—	0.5	5.0	4.2	—	—	5.4	3	—	—	0.1	0.2
Divorced and separated	—	—	0.4	—	—	—	—	—	1.1	0.2	—	—	—	—
Total	0.6	3.8	6.4	7.0	12.7	14.9	3.9	1.5	19.5	20.2	3.2	5.3	0.1	0.9

A = Family: mainly children, but also siblings, parents, etc. This includes indirect referrals to the Jewish Welfare Board, especially old-age homes applications; B = Neighbours and friends. Including social clubs and other day-care establishments; C = Hospitals: mainly as a means of achieving after-care therapy, but in many cases a way of ensuring that the patient receives adequate nourishment and other attention; D = Local authorities, social workers, community centres, district nurses, meals on wheels' staff and home helps; E = Jewish Welfare Board: previous connection with the organization or direct intervention by its social workers; F = Self-referrals: people who come across the Centre casually; G = Others: GP's, synagogues, charities and welfare organizations, etc.

for very short periods, utilizing it as a temporary refuge, providing meals and recreation.

A fair number of participants have become acquainted with the Centre through previous affiliation with the Jewish Welfare Board. Obviously for them the shame involved in any connection with the organization does not impede their association with the Centre. However, for the remaining 59.4 per cent of participants, this was a new trial.

As the formal criteria for admitting people to the Centre vary within the range of 'social isolation, physical handicap, inability to cope at home, the prevention of an explosive home situation getting out of hand by separation, ..., mental illness symptoms such as withdrawal, depression etc.',[1] the scope of eligibility is extremely broad. Loneliness and the inability to cope are the main motives for participation, but as they are both relative and personal they are open to endless interpretations. Since age is not a formal consideration, many members are younger than ought to be expected in a day centre for the elderly, and the age composition ranges from mid-forties to over-nineties.

TABLE 2.2 *Age structure in the Centre (in percentages), November 1974*

Under 50	50-59	60-69	70-79	80-89	90+	Total
1	3	27	50	18	1	100

Most of the younger participants are people suffering from mental disorders, slight retardation, or severe physical disabilities. Some of them are accompanied and attended by their parents or spouses. The presence of some younger people minimizes the impact of age as such on the image of the Centre, while the range of mental and physical handicaps constitute an added dimension to the heterogeneous nature of the participants.

In the absence of one prevailing attribute shared by all the participants, they cannot relate to each other according to a pre-existing common denominator. As people do not share the same problems, they cannot communicate and formulate norms and patterns of behaviour along the lines of these problems. The Centre is therefore an assemblage of people afflicted by various stigmas. These stigmas none the less provide a basis for mutual 'destigmatization'. All the participants are people who have been exposed to social rejection and avoidance, but this is the beginning and the end of the common ground between them.

The variety of personal handicaps and the age range play a major role in making the Centre a turning point in the participant's life, for here age, background, physical and mental disabilities – all factors which impinged on pre-Centre social life – lose their significance. This is because they are of little importance in establishing relationships with other people in the Centre. This is not to say that participants have reached the stage of ignoring and forgetting their plight, but it does indicate that these problems are no longer the hub of their lives. As one of the members pointed out to a newcomer, who complained about his health, accommodation and family situation, 'you are not going to impress anybody here, we are all experienced in this and you'd better start talking about interesting things.'

Distinctions in the Centre are created by other determinants, the physical structure of the premises being particularly significant. The two-storey building, a converted parish hall, comprises two large areas and very few small rooms. The lower floor is divided into six confined spaces, a kitchen, and a staff office overlooking a dining room-cum-recreation area furnished with tables and chairs, and equipped with a microphone, piano and sink unit. A removable partition separates it from an upper-level dark, oblong lounge, furnished with two opposing rows of armchairs, which serves as a working area and a sitting-room. It is adjacent to a small room – 'the rest room' – designed for the temporary seclusion for the sick or for small-scale meetings. This room adjoins a bath for the handicapped and a storage space for craft work and miscellaneous unused articles. Lavatories and a call box complete the structure of the ground floor.

The Centre entrance leads through a ramp to the dining area, and up two staircases to the upper floor. Here is a split-level, well-illuminated hall of which the larger, lower level is a working area and the narrower, upper level a stage. The hall is furnished with working tables and chairs and equipped with sewing machines, a reconditioned hundred-year-old printing machine, cupboards, and innumerable tools and materials which are scattered all over the place. There is also an office for craft teachers and a first-aid cabinet. A sink unit and lavatories lessen the need to go downstairs.

This structure, or rather what it lacks, has some significant

implications for the social life in the Centre. The fact that there is
no lift in the building presents an insuperable obstacle to severely
disabled people, especially those in wheelchairs or dependent on
walking frames or crutches, preventing them from taking advantage of the working area upstairs. Consequently, the lounge is
crammed with disabled people marooned in their armchairs, whereas the first floor is alive with more mobile participants, moving
around, engaging in craftwork, forming conversation circles,
exchanging jokes, and arguing.

As more disabled women than men attend the Centre, there is a
high proportion of women in the lounge, whereas men form the
majority on the upper floor (see 'Differentiations'). This imbalance
further marks the difference between the two areas. The image of
'old crones' chattering away, moaning and grumbling, languishing
in the lounge is opposed to the image of vigorous, creative 'boys'
labouring upstairs.

Two fire exits connect the two floors, but although they are at
the disposal of the participants they are very rarely used, despite the
congestion of the main staircase leading from the entrance. One
cannot escape the impression that negotiating the stairs has become
a valued sign of mobility and physical fitness, by which a person
qualifies as a member of the most highly esteemed category of
participants. Thus one can often observe people standing seemingly
aimlessly on the stairs, or trying to initiate a conversation whilst
lingering on their way up or down.

Apart from the two offices, the 'rest room' and the toilets, there
are no sanctuaries in the Centre to which people can retreat for a
while, to escape the hustle and bustle in the large undivided spaces.
Participants are perpetually exposed to uncontrolled contact. The
constant movement makes the immediate physical and social environment unstable and rather casual. The only way to overcome this
lack of privacy is to confine oneself to an armchair and to switch
off. This needs determination, for others are quick to insinuate
lack of sociability, and there are constant invitations to take part in
conversation, work and recreational activity.

This shifting character of the environment is accentuated by the
functional versatility of the available space. No elaborate work or
sophisticated entertainment, requiring special equipment, takes
place in the Centre, and so the same space may be used for various
purposes. Thus the dining hall is a place of entertainment, and the

craft and keep-fit classes meet there. It provides a place for discussions, general meetings, talks and staff meetings, and it is also, of course, a dining hall. The lounge is a rest area as well as a working area, and the upstairs hall, with its stage and miscellaneous furniture, serves various groups and enterprises. Decisions concerning the use of any space are a function of the daily routine and services offered by the Centre, and the relationship between staff and participants, and between participants themselves. The behavioural aspect of the Centre will be discussed at some length later, but a brief account of the structure and the daily operation of the establishment will complete this outline.

The Jewish Welfare Board's Marlsden team comprises two units,[2] the field-workers and the Centre staff. Three social workers visit clients and act as a channel between them and the services available from the Board. The Centre staff itself consists of twelve people, including two full time drivers, three kitchen staff (a cook and two assistants), one craft assistant, a general assistant, a social organizer, an administrative assistant, one social worker, a deputy supervisor (until November 1974) and a supervisor. This is in addition to two cleaners and craft and keep-fit instructors from the Inner London Education Authority. Only the supervisor, his deputy and the social workers possess some qualifications in social work. The rest are not trained social workers, and came to the Centre from various walks of life. The turnover amongst staff is fairly high and during the year of research only the administrative assistant, the craft assistant, the cooks and one of the drivers remained at their posts.

The Centre is open from 9.00 a.m. to 5.00 p.m. from Monday to Thursday, and on most Sunday afternoons. On Friday mornings the participants go to the Jewish Blind Society's day centre along with the JBS members.[3] Apart from special occasions, like festivals or outings, participants attend whenever they like, and with the exception of lunch-time and tea-time, there are no rules about attendance.

Most of the participants arrive by bus, using their free bus passes, and alighting a very short distance from the building. However, transport is provided for the severely handicapped. This arrangement is described by the organizers:[4]

'Both our drivers make two "collections" and corresponding

"deliveries" per day. The first coaches start to pick up the participants at 8.30 a.m., and these people are taken home from
1.45 p.m.

The second coach rounds commence at 10.45 a.m., and these
participants are taken back from the Centre around 3.00 p.m.
Apart from wheelchair cases, people brought in by transport
suffer from disabilities including the usual range of those associated with old age – osteo-arthritis, cardiac conditions etc.

Perhaps the most crucial, frustrating and sensitive area of
operations for the staff is the transporting of handicapped and
less mobile participants to and from the Centre. The tail-lift
ambulance and the Ford Transit coach call for tact, anticipation, and invariably an element of luck. Accommodating the
particular demands of some 140 participants whose attendance,
once to four times weekly, is often unpredictable, and whose
ability to co-operate with simple routines is unreliable, proves to
be a daily headache. At the same time "transport" embraces the
addition of new names from the waiting list to those being
currently transported: I suppose some 5 or 6 new applications
for coach places reach us each month.

We must constantly remember that we are taking aged and
disabled pensioners to and from the Day Centre, not inanimate
consignments of cargo. Perhaps the most confusing and haras-
sing aspect is the gathering of data and information about
members' movements, their (often) unyielding expectations, and
selfish requests for priority.

"Juggling" would be an apt term to apply to the daily task of
preparing the drivers' lists. We attempt to utilize all the space
available in both coaches (two rounds each morning) matching
transport "cases" with the capacity of the coaches. Mistakes
occasionally occur either because messages go adrift, are mis-
understood or because the markers on the transport wall-chart
are accidentally disturbed. Many other unpredictable factors
upset the most carefully laid plans.

Vacant coach spaces (like gold dust) are a rarity and we
attempt to place those waiting in some sort of priority order. But
I am conscious of the need to be elastic – emergency (direct)
hospital referrals for example must have an obvious priority. We
must constantly avoid over-reacting to moral blackmail etc., for
the sake of running the system as fairly as possibly. ...'

As most of the organized social activities held in the Centre take place after lunch, almost all the transport people are precluded from participating in them. This exclusion, added to their other limitations, means that their attendance is restricted to very few contacts and engagements in the Centre.

Catering in the Centre is a second sensitive area between staff and participants. Some of the problems are outlined by a member of staff:[5]

'By the end of July 1974 the Day Centre was providing up to 140 daily meals from Monday to Thursday, as well as morning and afternoon teas. Although accurate comparative statistics cannot be given for the whole year, there was no appreciable reduction in the number of meals served when meal charges of 10p were introduced in early February,[6] and these now run at 120 participants (average) per day, 9 staff and 10–15 voluntary and paid kitchen staff: lunches are served in two sittings.

Originally the cook and kitchen assistants were preparing no more than 100 hot meals each day. They have now raised the number by about 40 per cent to absorb newcomers since early this year, but this has not been without its difficulties. The provision of three separate diets – ordinary, gastric and diabetic – was accomplished by virtue of careful meal planning and preparations. But the strain became evident and so it was recently decided to discontinue gastric diets since the system was in any event being abused by a small number of members. We found that there were, in some instances, no valid medical reasons for an individual to adhere to a gastric diet; genuine cases however are still provided with a salad or omelette meal. The steep rise in numbers placed an ever-increasing emotional and physical strain on the staff.

The role of the volunteer helpers at lunches has proved to be very important. On the whole they have carried out dining-room support duties with the minimum of fuss and direction. Small problems could more accurately be described as misunderstandings. The benefits and advantages of volunteers' assistance at the Centre far outweigh the so-called shortcomings. Without them meal-time order could by now have descended into chaos.

The seating capacity of the dining room (about 80) is such that the entire area becomes extremely crowded during the lunch period. Controlling this potential hazard as people move in and out (up and down the ramp) is never easy and one or two members of staff are required to watch these movements. Pressures upon the staff are perhaps greatest at these times, and the "policing" is never really adequate. One of the causes of the difficulty is the crowding of the ramp area before first-sitting lunch and then immediately before the second sitting when the tables are being relaid.'

The distribution of participants between the two sittings is normally regulated by the tendency of the disabled in the lounge to attend the first sitting and for the upstairs people to go to the second. This is due to a combination of two factors. As most of the disabled are dependent on transport, they have to prepare themselves for the journey home as soon as the drivers finish their meal, which leaves them with very little time to get ready. The people upstairs do not face this problem. The second factor, which follows from the first, is that attending the later sitting distinguishes one from those who attend the first sitting. These people are not only handicapped, but they are also regarded by the upstairs people as parasites, taking advantage of the Centre's services without contributing towards its activities.

Although attendance indicates material difficulties, the Centre is not looked upon as a communal kitchen, or a luncheon club. The sense of belonging to the place reaches far beyond the services it provides (see 'Boundaries'). Any member who denies this widely accepted postulate, by coming to the Centre just for his lunch, represents a threat to the whole foundation of participation. These people are publicly rebuked, disparaged, and complained about to staff. The concept of participation is a complex edifice, constructed from relationships with the outside world in addition to the activities in the Centre. Relationships with the outside world will be discussed in the section on boundaries, but the daily activities in the Centre may be sketched here.

A regular morning activity is craft work. In the words of a member of staff:[7]

'The Centre from its original inception has always followed a policy of trying to involve participants in craft work for its therapeutic and creative value.

We have an ILEA lecturer, who is at the Centre four days a

week. In addition, ILEA supply the following:

Dressmaking instructress	– once weekly
Soft furnishing teacher	– once weekly
Keep fit teacher (accompanied by pianist)	– twice weekly
2 general crafts instructresses	– twice weekly
1 general crafts instructress	– once weekly
Beauty care instructress	– twice weekly
Musical appreciation	– once weekly

General crafts include cane-work, mosaic, patchwork, rug making, knitting, crochet, soft toy making, collage, stool making etc.

We have been hit during the year by staff shortages and this has affected craft work to a large extent. There is a need for qualified people to help out and the brunt of the burden has had to be borne by elderly participants on the ground floor, who are possibly more restricted in the type of work that they can do. More handicapped members require much patience and often skill and very few teachers are able to take them on. Such members are possibly less responsive and less rewarding in their output than their more able fellow participants. As a consequence the brunt of the work has fallen on Day Centre staff already fully stretched in attending to supervisory duties, group activities and to individual social work.

We feel that this is a difficult state of affairs, but since we do not have direct control over ILEA staff, there is little we can do at present to ease the situation. We are also hampered by lack of storage space within the Centre, in particular, lack of cupboards and wardrobes to store textiles, materials and finished articles. There have been difficulties with the delivery of certain materials and equipment necessary to craft work. There have been big delays in deliveries and quite often when materials do arrive, they are of the wrong kind and do not correspond to the materials ordered.'

Conflicts with ILEA staff exist on several fronts:[8]

'In general there has been a conflict in the conception of "craft work" between the ILEA and ourselves. The ILEA think in terms of "classes", presumably in a controlled quiet room, isolated, where the tutor can expect the ready co-operation of his "students". This obviously is not so at our Centre with its big halls and bustling interaction of participants. There are always going to be minor crises and distractions to disrupt the concentration of both participants and tutors. We feel that the Centre is engaged in craft work, first and foremost as a therapeutic exercise, whereas the ILEA tutors tend to look to the standard of the work produced. It seems to us that if people are occupied in work which is of relative interest, we should not concern ourselves too much with trying to produce individual work of a very high standard, although, of course, we are pleased when this does occur. As a consequence, I feel that by concentrating on small groups of people only, who are capable of a high standard of work, the ILEA tutors are trying to impose a work atmosphere which is not suitable for the Centre. The result is that we are left with the brunt of the work in trying to keep the bulk of our participants interested in craft work, and we have felt the strain throughout the year. I feel that the ILEA staff should increase the scope of their work to cover people who are not so capable or interested. These participants must be *made* to feel interested, i.e. we and the ILEA staff *must go out* to them rather than expect them to come to us. In other words, tutors should be more *adaptable* to our type of atmosphere and should be more *available* to a larger group of people.'

This ideology of the 'appropriate approach' towards participants is practised in the running of the Centre, which will be discussed separately, but it also manifests itself in other aspects of Centre activities.

Participants are free to use the amplification systems for their own entertainment. They are also at liberty to arrange discussion groups, to hold meetings, and in general to take initiatives in any recreational area so long as they do not clash with lunch and transport arrangements. This freedom is taken full advantage of, and singing, dancing, bingo, and raffle draws are organized by participants. Regular and organized control of these activities is made possible by the operation of a committee of participants sponsored by a fund – 'The Benevolent Fund' – to which weekly contributions are made. The functions of the committee in relation to staff are ill-defined and a potential area for conflicts and disputes. From the staff point of view, the benevolent fund[9]

'was set up to meet a real need. The Jewish Welfare Board made it clear that they could not finance certain activities which were thought peripheral to the actual running of the Centre. For example, the financing of outings and of visits to members in hospital. It also enabled a bridging of the gap between the staff and members to create a dialogue. The committee at present comprises some 15 members, all of whom undertake some executive duties. It is chaired by the supervisor and consists of a weekly contribution of 3p by all members, which is collected and recorded by committee members. The Treasurer is a committee member. This fund raising has stimulated other projects, such as raffles, sales of clothing and independent contributions, as well as a dance last March. In the first six months of the operation of the fund, nearly £200 was collected from contributions and slightly more than this amount from other sources mentioned. The summer has seen two seaside trips catering for 106 participants per time and wholly organized by committee members. A trip to a country house for 26 handicapped participants and to Westcliff for 70, including 15 chairbound persons and involving five coaches. All of this has been done independently of the Board.

In addition, committee members have helped the staff in various ways. The completion of the register, serving, distributions and washing up of lunches, the collection of lunch monies, the organization of social activities are increasingly being undertaken by participants themselves.'

The function of the committee as seen by some of its members is, however, more far-reaching and comprehensive. They expect to be recognized as taking an equal share with staff in the management of the Centre. The 'executive duties' delegated to them by staff, such as keeping order at lunch times, collecting money and keeping the register of daily attendances at the entrance hall have provided opportunities for them to assume further responsibilities, such as admitting new participants, and hence to claim more power and authority.

Discords and contentions amongst committee members are a daily occurrence. A few co-operate with staff in attempting to restrain fellow committee members, while others try to initiate activities under their own steam, to enhance their influence. Occasional general meetings in which the participants meet with the committee allow these internal conflicts to be aired in public. Accusations and counter-accusations are exchanged, and there is evident an awareness and concern about the position and the activities of members of the committee, and the ways in which they handle the affairs of the participants (see 'Patterns of Help').

Other activities are organized in part or wholly by the staff. In some instances they liaise between participants and outside guests – speakers, entertainers, etc. Other events are organized and conducted entirely by staff. These include discussion groups, sales, talks, announcements, craft work, art classes, etc. Attendance is usually high and very rarely is it necessary to persuade people to participate. What is particularly striking is the number of discussions and debates organized by a few members of staff, and the extent to which they are looked forward to by participants.

Activities in the Centre, though containing a strong repetitive element, do not follow set patterns. Activities are dropped, renovated, and their form and content changed, but within parameters set by attitudes to time, and to participation, which will be dealt with later on. However, certain changes are due to factors which are beyond the control of participants: following decisions taken at an official level, caused by staff turnover, even influenced by development in local government policies. It would be a distortion to present the history of the Centre without regard to the reaction of its participants, but certain developments are immune from the participants' influence.

The Centre was set up in 1970, after a survey carried out by the Jewish Welfare Board into the conditions of the aged Jewish population of Marlsden. It shared its premises with another club, and this hampered its activities. The attendance was 10–15 people a day, 2–3 times a week. In fact, in facilities and membership it resembled a friendship club (with a communal kitchen). Participants were not asked to pay for their meals, their bus fares were reimbursed and they even earned some money by engaging in light industrial work.

In 1972 the Board purchased an old parish hall for the new premises of the Centre. The move was accompanied by organizational changes, and caused a flow of newcomers who found the new, spacious environment less restrictive, and more responsive to their needs. The free bus pass for the elderly resulted in the cancellation of reimbursed fares, forcing participants to watch their return time carefully, as after 4.00 p.m. this concession is not valid. Lunches and teas ceased to be free of charge, initially as a therapeutic measure designed to eliminate the feeling of living on charity, and thus to boost feelings of independence and self-respect. Later, the money raised in this way became a significant source of revenue, and charges have nearly tripled in a matter of three years. Although not welcomed, this move did not cause particular outrage amongst participants, who accepted the rationale given by staff to justify the rises.

Industrial work has continued, but its popularity and weight in Centre life is on the decline. This work includes assembling, packing, etc. and the income is no longer paid to the individual participants, but to the Centre. Members of staff commented:[10]

> 'Whilst realizing that it is possibly more rewarding and creative to interest the participants in craft work, we feel that there will always be room in the Centre for industrial work to cater for those (a) who are incapable of concentrating for long periods of time on craft work, and (b) those who feel that craft work is really not "serious" enough for them to become interested in or "too feminine". Such work simulates a real work situation for many members who insist on every one pulling their weight. There is keen interest in how much money is earned.'

However, participants periodically call for the reintroduction of personal payment. These requests are carefully discussed, but have been dismissed by members of staff on the grounds that the Centre is not a workshop, and should not be regarded as merely a working place.

The year of fieldwork in the Centre commenced at the end of May 1974 and was completed at the beginning of July 1975. This period was marked by changes in two areas. The first concerns the relationship of the Centre with the Jewish Blind Society, and the second relates to changes in staffing and authority in the Centre.

The decision to establish a link between the Jewish Welfare Board and the Jewish Blind Society was taken in headquarters as a result of interorganizational policies concerning the distribution of funds between Jewish charities. It was felt that a possible merger between the two organizations would produce a better utilization of communal resources. As the Jewish Blind Society administers a day centre for the blind and partially sighted nearby, an experimental link was arranged, with the sharing of premises and facilities once a week.

Under this scheme, the participants of the Centre went or were transported every Friday to the modern, spacious, well-equipped and under-utilized Jewish Blind Society day centre. The difference in regime and staff attitudes made it impossible to transfer the Centre atmosphere and activities to the new environment, and the reaction to this weekly shift ranged from indifference to resentment. As tension between participants from the two day centres grew, a new step was decided upon. Every other week the members of the Jewish Blind Society would attend the Centre.

The staff opposed this step and complied reluctantly. As discord and complaints increased, it was suggested that a third stage in the project be implemented. This entailed the separation of the able-bodied and disabled ('transport people'). The former would be transferred every Friday to the Jewish Blind Society, whilst the latter would continue to be catered for at the Centre. Participants and staff alike objected strongly but had to accept the arrangement, though regarding it as a set-back to their hopes for the Centre community.

These significant changes were outside the control of the participants. Another factor they cannot control is the turnover amongst staff, particularly that caused by changes in organization in head office. During the year of fieldwork two resignations, one dismissal, one secondment leave, two transfers and five new appointments took place, of which the most important was the change of supervisor.

Until the middle of 1975, the area team of Marlsden was divided into two separate units – the fieldworkers and the Centre staff – headed by two leaders of equal rank. A new post of area team leader was created, and the supervision of the Centre from its inception was selected for it. This necessitated a replacement in the Centre, and, following a lengthy selection process, the new supervisor took charge.

It is always difficult to handle personalities in a sociological discussion, but the differences between these two supervisors underlies their respective approaches to the Centre as well as the reactions they provoked. The first supervisor was a thirty-one-year-old, qualified social worker who had almost no experience outside the Centre. His replacement, who took office from mid January 1975, was a

sixty-four-year-old retired businessman, who had no training as a
social worker but who had engaged in community work. They
contrasted in many ways, but probably the most significant
contrast lay between the emphasis on organization and order of the
second supervisor and the policy of involvement and informality of
his predecessor. The implications of this contrast will emerge as I
describe the running of the Centre in more detail.

The running of the Centre

To analyse the Centre as an arena of power and authority would be
a futile exercise unless one contrasted this with a model of the
Centre as an environment 'caring' for the elderly, an approach
which reveals different if not opposite characteristics. Such a comparison brings out the unique features of the Centre, and suggests
an approach to the variations in old people's behaviour under
different systems. The obvious alternative to a day centre is an old
age home, and this comparison will be invoked from time to time.[11]

The fact that the Centre is not a total environment covering all
aspects of life and providing a comprehensive service throughout
the day, in turn limits the participants' dependence on Centre services. They may choose to use the Centre as a cheap communal
kitchen, a recreation place, both or neither. They may attend whenever they wish and make their own personal balance between the
amount of time and degree of involvement invested in the Centre
and that devoted to their autonomous lives outside it. Although
pressures by staff as well as by participants to partake in as many
Centre activities as possible do exist, the decision is still left to the
individual and there is no coercion. Moreover, since attendance is
irregular, participants are not required and, indeed, cannot be
asked to commit themselves to conform to an agenda laid down for
them by staff. Nor can groups count on particular participants.
Thus, certain discussion groups are based on the regular attendance
of some articulate and interested participants, but their attendance
is unpredictable, and in their absence the meetings dissolve.

This lack of firm rules and regulations is recognized by participants, and statements such as 'everybody can do whatever he likes
here', or, 'nobody can compel us to do this' are common, particularly with respect to choosing when to attend. Nevertheless, there
are three areas in which some sort of order and restraint must be

operated. These are transport arrangements, lunch sittings, and social work, all rendering a direct service to participants and involving the allocation of certain resources amongst them, and all provoking conflict and power struggles.

Transport is the front for two battles, the first engaging people who consider themselves eligible for the service, and who try to push their way into a place on the daily rounds; and the second involving participants who already enjoy the service, but express their independence of it by deliberately disturbing its smooth running.

Applying for a place on the 'transport list' takes various forms, ranging from quiet pleading to barging onto the coach. The transport organizer has to sustain constant pressure accompanied by threats, tears and continuous nagging. However, the brunt of the pressure is often on the drivers, who are subjected to direct approaches by participants who are caught up in circumstances like temporary immobility, bad weather, etc. The power of the driver is accentuated by the fact that in the absence of an escort to the coaches he is expected to help his passengers in and out, to deal with emergencies, and to see that they all reach their residence safely.

This is not an easy job to carry out, particularly considering the contrary behaviour of some of the passengers. This manifests itself in long delays caused by participants who linger over dressing and preparing themselves, purposely wasting time as a means of asserting their power and autonomy. Apart from hooting and shouting there is very little the driver can do to hurry these people up, and he cannot use sanctions against them. The result is that the timetable for the rounds is disturbed and conflict between drivers and their passengers is chronic.

Another area in which clashes between staff and participants are unavoidable is in the organization of lunch. This also provides people with an opportunity to defy authority and proclaim independence. As there is no menu to choose from, there is ample scope for expressing dissatisfaction with the food, the way it is served, and the inevitable differences in sizes of portions. Since lunch is chargeable, participants feel that they are entitled to their opinions. Some complaints led to open rows between participants and staff, and between the participants themselves. The two additional diets which are often claimed and obtained by non-eligible participants complicate matters considerably.

Another aspect of lunch time is the inadequate seating capacity of the dining hall. During the two overcrowded sittings people are fighting over places and jumping the queue. Consequently disciplinary measures have to be imposed and members of staff take turns in guarding the ramp and supervising the orderly distribution of participants between the two sessions. As this arrangement did not prevent the pre-emption of seats, the undisciplined barging into the hall, the participants' help was sought. Members of the committee were asked to regulate the stream of participants heading towards the hall from the lounge and down the stairs. This move provoked defiance and fierce objections. Very few participants were inclined to recognize this delegation of authority as legitimate. An attempt was made by members of the committee, at the request of staff, to block the main door of the upper floor, to prevent people from running down the stairs to seize seats before lunch time was announced through the loudspeakers. Although participants knew there were two fire escapes leading to the dining hall, nobody tried to evade control by using them. Instead, they preferred to throng by the main door, argue with the 'wardens', and force their way downstairs.

Members of staff threatened to stop serving lunch altogether. A system of allocation priorities according to severity of disablement was tried. Each move was foiled by the intractable participants, who made it their goal to prevent lunch time from reflecting a style of dependency characteristic of an old-age home. The image of life in such a home and its ominous predecessor – the workhouse – haunts participants and, as will be shown later, they will do anything they can to prevent its shadow falling on the Centre.

A more complicated area of allocating resources involves the social worker employed on the premises. The initiative to apply to this social worker is left to the participants, as not every participant is automatically in need of a social worker's attention and, therefore, 'although social workers are employed at the Centre they maintain a low profile'.[12] The social worker commented:[13]

'Although my official title is "Social Worker", one of the first things I realized when I came to work at the Centre, is that nobody's role is clearly defined, and consequently social work is often neglected for other duties necessitated by the every-day running of the Centre.

I would describe the type of social work done at the Centre as "informal", inasmuch as there are no interviewing rooms and no particular times set aside for the participants to discuss their problems with the social workers. This situation is, of course, far from ideal as it is very difficult to find the time or the place to sit down for any length of time and talk to a participant without being interrupted, and I would say that we can only hope to touch the surface of people's problems.

The main problem that every participant shares is one of loneliness, but the majority of the problems that I am approached to help with are usually stereotyped domestic problems which only require a letter or a telephone call. The amount of grants made at the Centre is gradually lessening as the emphasis is on helping the participants to help themselves rather than being dependent on others.

As a direct result of lack of individual attention given to the participants, a lot of emphasis has been on group work, e.g. discussions, rather than concentrating on particular individuals, which is carried out by the Day Centre staff in general.'

The impression that the Centre is moulded by the participants' initiatives is created not only by the form of social work done there, but also by the way members of staff perform their roles in the Centre. The Centre staff, being part of the Marlsden team, occupy themselves mainly with the relationship of participants with the outside environment, especially with services and problems concerning their general welfare. This is done in conjunction with the fieldworkers, partly at weekly 'allocation meetings' held in the Centre. The staff is involved in the lives of participants outside the Centre, visiting members at home, helping with everyday difficulties and giving advice on personal problems as well as relationships with social welfare agencies. The emphasis on the extra-institutional lives of the participants presents a sharp contrast to the situation in a home for the aged. This relates to another relevant contrast, in the structure of hierarchy amongst staff.

The conventional view of authority structures in total institutions is of a pyramid with well defined echelons, embracing all aspects of institutional life. Nothing of the sort exists in the Centre. Although the supervisor[14] is formally in charge of the running of the Centre, and very little control is exerted by head office, there is no system of authority delegation, or even a defined role structure. It is significant that participants are usually unable to point out any formal differences between staff, viewing them mainly as individuals. Every member of staff fulfils various interchangeable functions, determined mainly by circumstances. The supervisor refused to set up barriers on the model of the boss-employee relationship. Staff should not expect him to make all the decisions, but should be prepared to assume full responsibility for the way they perform their jobs. This approach stems both from the organizational position of the supervisor as the only mediator co-ordinating the relations between head office, the fieldworkers and the Centre staff, and from his general conception of social work and staff-participant relationships.

The supervisor who replaced him was directly accountable to him in his new capacity of area team leader of Marlsden. The new man was carefully watched and advised, and had almost no direct dealings with head office. It is interesting that the new supervisor tried to introduce a system of authority much closer in nature to the stereotype one would expect to find within a bureaucratic setting. As his responsibility was strictly confined to the running of the Centre he endeavoured to consolidate and safeguard his control over staff, detaching them from their previous allegiances to the Marlsden team and from their involvement with the participants in their lives outside the Centre. This process initiated a rudimentary transformation of the Centre from a system channelling its resources outward, into a more segregated, self-contained unit, more inward-looking and more concerned with its own structure. Thus members of staff were asked to produce weekly reports on their work, to lay down a detailed programme of planned activities, publicized on the Centre notice board, and to concentrate on organizing their own formally designated field. Staff meetings, which had formerly been characterized by loose agendas, occasional small-talk, and which were even informal 'therapy groups', became an arena for role definitions and the inception of a distinct vertical hierarchy.

This process of establishing a strict division of labour between members of staff initiated a process of disengagement from the participants. The first sign of this was the unsuccessful attempt to abolish the category of volunteers. These are participants' wives and other non-participants who find it fulfilling and rewarding to help in the Centre, mainly in serving lunch and tea. They are highly integrated with the participants, and in fact it is rather hard to tell a volunteer from an active participant. This hybrid between an unpaid worker and a participant, of doubtful identity but exercising authority, presented a potential threat to the new system. Only the fact that serving lunch would have been almost impossible without the help of these volunteers prevented their dismissal.

This observation suggests another contrast between the Centre under the first supervisor and a conventional old age home. This concerns the staff–client dichotomy. In some total institutions there appears to be an unbridgeable gap between the two, engendered by the staff's conception of the clients as objects of care and handling. This attitude was not developed among staff at the Centre. Relationships with participants were based on the expectation, inculcated by the supervisor and supported by most members of staff, that clients should be involved, should participate.

The concept of participation stems from the premise that the facilities and amenities provided by the Centre are not nearly sufficient for the clients' needs. Their problems are seen as arising fundamentally from loneliness and depression. The clients need companionship and empathy. To achieve this, members of staff must overcome barriers of sex, age, authority, education and background. They must aim at a full identification with the participant's thoughts and feelings, an acceptance of his conception of the world, in order to share his problems with him and try to alleviate them.

This attitude manifests itself in informal relationships with participants; in an 'open door' policy which admits anybody to the Centre simply on the grounds that he wants to join it; in participating in the participants' activities, and not only by organizing and instructing. An ideal member of staff, according to the supervisor, is one who assimilates himself completely into the participants' world but as a stimulant. This depends on personality and the emotional investment a member of staff is willing to make. In practice, it entails disregard of official working hours, involving members of the family in the Centre activities, and the obliteration of role definition whilst dealing with participants.

The naked reality that members of staff are not participants, do not share the same problems, come from different environments and backgrounds, and look upon their jobs as a means of living, inevitably creates disagreements, opposition and intrigue amongst staff. Two cases will illustrate the difficulties of the policy.

Rose was an unqualified general assistant doing miscellaneous jobs, moving around briskly, ubiquitous, chatting away, helping and organizing. The occasional visitor would undoubtedly get the impression that Rose was an active participant. In late middle-age, she dressed, talked and behaved like a participant. One could hardly tell the difference. Rose lived in the area, was already acquainted with a great number of participants, and possessed extensive knowledge of their lives and backgrounds. The fact that Rose's husband was the senior driver of the Centre provided an additional dimension to her involvement with the participants. She was regarded by her fellow staff members as 'an extension of the participants, who just happened to get paid' and therefore, as the supervisor put it, 'an indispensable asset to the Centre', representing the epitome of his participation approach. Rose herself accepted this position, but not without problems and reservations.

Rose invited participants to her house, discussed her personal problems with them, and even tried to involve them in her financial affairs. But she became concerned with what she regarded as the intrusion of the Centre into her private life, and the effect of this on her family. During the period of fieldwork she was constantly vacillating between leaving the Centre or staying. This was accompanied by her recurrent attempts to redefine her position by setting up barriers between herself and the participants, and delineating the area of her involvement with the Centre life.

She concentrated her effort on two targets. Members of staff used to lunch together in the second sitting, and it was impossible to prevent participants either from choosing to sit at their table, or from interrupting the meal by asking for help and advice. Most members of staff, although obviously disturbed by this behaviour, showed no overt signs of distress or anger, and tried to remain composed. Rose, on the other hand, raged at the interrupters, shouted them down, and made it clear that there was no place for participants at the staff table.

Her aggressive insistence on her position as a staff member was also expressed in her relationships with the volunteers – like her, intermediate between staff and participants. Being served by them at lunch, she took this opportunity to make her position as a member of staff as evident as possible to them. This was done by ordering them about, asking for services not usually provided, and taking charge and supervising the service. The altercations this behaviour provoked helped Rose to assert her status in the eyes of watching participants, but did not contribute to her establishing herself as an equal member of staff in the view of her colleagues.

Rose then insisted on a review of her job definition, with the intention of investing it with greater prestige. She was not satisfied with the title of 'general assistant', or 'day-centre attendant' as she was termed in the Centre records. There was no official ground for this application and it was refused. After further resignation threats and ominous absences, Rose left the Centre for good.

Whereas Rose was trying to avoid complete identification with participants, Joan found herself accused of remoteness and uninvolvement. Twenty-one years old, an ex-model and a Gentile, Joan could hardly be classified as a typical participant, and her view of the appropriate relationship between staff and participants only increased the distance. Joan maintained that a distinct line should be drawn between her work in the Centre and her private life. She, therefore, refused to answer participants' queries concerning her private life, and made it quite clear to the staff that, apart from special occasions, she would not stay in the Centre for any longer than the official working hours. Furthermore, she asked that in her dealings with participants she should be directed by the supervisor, and that a clear definition of roles and authority should be introduced.

This attitude incensed some members of staff and provoked arguments and recriminations. Basically Joan was accused of not fulfilling the expected function of a staff member. She did not invest her whole personality and feelings into the job. Joan pleaded in return that, although she acted as a friend to the participants, she could not see the Centre as the hub of her life.

Nevertheless, a few months after her admission Joan gradually intensified her involvement and her insistence on working according to the rules weakened. As she herself said, 'I am becoming like Rose – a perfect participant.' The forces which engulfed Joan, as well as other members of staff, are part of the overall atmosphere of the Centre and will be discussed later.

These two contrary tendencies, to participation or withdrawal, could be recognized to varying degrees in the behaviour of all members of staff, although differences arose due to personal and structural factors. Thus, the administrative assistant who was confined to the office most of the day and had, therefore, little direct contact with participants, could not and indeed did not wish to involve herself more deeply than required for the proper performance of her duties. One of the craft assistants, one driver and the cook were in similar situations. All of these had better defined roles than other members, which may account for the differences in approach.

The 'participation' policy did not eliminate altogether the differences between staff and participants and, therefore, did not guarantee a harmonious relationship between them. This was inevitable given the resources in the hands of the staff, and the realization by participants that, despite the 'participation' approach, there was a fundamentally unbridgeable gap, perceived in terms of careers and time, rather than in terms of power and roles. Participants were fully conscious of the fact that members of staff, however devoted to the Centre and good at their jobs, were still passers-by in the establishment, which was a training ground or a stage through which they advanced in their careers. Furthermore, there was the awareness that the lives of members of staff centred around their families and the external environment. This presented a sharp contrast to the 'Centre-centred' participant – a contrast which was sometimes regarded unfavourably and even with resentment.

Some participants handled the consequent ambivalence by 'obliterating' the presence of staff as such, even though physically and formally, of course, the people concerned remained unaffected. Thus some participants insisted that most members of staff spent their day in the office doing paper work, although actually that crammed room could hardly accommodate more than four people standing, let alone sitting down. These participants maintained that 'the Centre runs itself', and that the staff was an unnecessary nuisance. As Alan, one of the leading spokesmen, put it 'The Centre is so successful because we are nice people – friendly and helpful – it has got nothing to do with the staff.' He also added that there was no doubt in his mind that, given the opportunity, the participants would run the Centre better than the staff. They would extend activities in the evenings, install an elevator to enable better integration, and show more concern for the participants' problems outside. He accused staff of not having the Centre's interests at heart, and of using it merely to promote their own position in the head office of the organization.

Direct confrontations were averted by the fact that most members of staff were busy on the ground floor, aiding the handicapped, preparing lunches, and holding discussion groups, keep-fit classes and other activities. The upper hall, therefore, remained a staff-free territory, and apart from the ILEA instructors and the craft assistant, there was only one member of staff in an organizing capacity in charge of the whole floor. During the field-work period two people filled that function in succession, and both made significant adjustments to the role allocated to them by participants. The first, an unqualified social worker, identified himself with the participants to the extent of sitting with them, doing craft work and engaging in small talk and gossip. He developed personal friendships with a number of them, inviting them to his home and seeing to their problems in a manner which went far beyond his duties as a member of staff. In staff meetings he invariably supported the participants' views and opposed any move to monitor or supervise their activities. The participants themselves saw him as an uprooted person (being a bachelor immigrant from New Zealand, with no relations or affiliations in England) who had no other career but the Centre and who, therefore, was in the same position as they were.

His replacement, Joan, being determined to separate her private life from her job, was at first ignored by the participants, and later subjected to snide remarks, such as 'go and make the tea, you are not good for anything else'. (Making the tea is an accepted task of the volunteers.) In one participant's view, 'Joan is good only for one thing ... and I wouldn't mind doing it with her.'

The variations in staff participation do not, however, reflect the general conception of the participants which actually prevails amongst staff. Fundamentally, they regard participants as people who have ceased to think for themselves, resist and fear change, and enjoy a predictable, controllable environment offering no excitement or purpose. As the supervisor described them, they are 'ritual people as opposed to drama people'. This approach, corresponding to the one suggested in 'The end of involvement', is supported by the impression given by participants' attitudes towards the Centre. They tend to see it as a bounded unit, set off from the outside world, in which events have no effect outside, and are not impinged upon by outside circumstances.[15] This view of the Centre leads to a series of questions concerning the boundaries delineating the Centre.

Boundaries

Two complementary groups of factors define the boundaries setting off the Centre from its surroundings. The first includes environmental determinants, all of which, being beyond the Centre's
manipulation, are merely responded to by participants. The second
derives from the world of the Centre, and affect and mark the
relationships with the outside world.

'Losing face' because of entering the Centre is a factor which
should not be underestimated in considering the barriers between
the participants and the outside world. Irrespective of their truth,
judgments like 'you must be really hard up to go to the Centre',
and, 'no wonder that people point you out and whisper', are widespread amongst participants, and indicate their overriding realization that they are regarded with disdain and pity, as social misfits
who have failed to fend for themselves, and, therefore, become the
clients of a charity. Other elderly Jews in the Marlsden community
do indeed look down on participation in the Centre. Attending the
Centre implies inadequate income and hence a low financial position as well as an inability to command family support. Old people
not far removed from this state make every effort to disassociate
themselves from the Centre participants. Thus, two participants
who decided to get married in the local synagogue encountered
rejection and something like contempt on their wedding day from
their elderly contemporaries who comprised the local congregation.
A married couple in their late seventies, who were confronted by
most of the hardships attributed to the Centre people, adamantly
refused even to pay a visit to the place as 'we are decent people, not
paupers and we will never mingle with that lot'.

This awareness of rejection and indignity is accentuated by the
scarcity of visits and indications of concern from individuals and
organizations in the area. Apart from one or two visits by local
politicians – mainly as a canvassing attempt in election campaigns –
or the occasional representative of some association or public
service, the Centre is of no interest to the community. One of the
reasons for this is, perhaps, its denominational tag. To quote one
of the social workers:[16]

'The relationship between the Day Centre and the community as
a whole is rather difficult to define as many agencies in the area
remain unaware of our existence whilst others feel that whilst a

Day Centre catering for the elderly and handicapped is, of course, beneficial and greatly needed, it goes against the grain of many Local Authority Social Workers to refer their clients to a Centre where the main criterion for entry is to be of the Jewish faith.'

This was further elaborated on by the supervisor:[17]

'There is clearly a feeling in the Social Service hierarchy that the Jewish community is well able to look after its own, or perhaps should look after its own. Also various members of staff have come up against the prevailing social work ethos amongst the younger graduate or newly qualified Social Worker that the task of Social Services is to integrate the whole community and that denominational organizations militate against this. It is likely that some go as far as to ignore the presence of the Centre in dealing with Jewish people.'

Except for the Jewish Blind Society and the Jewish Home and Hospital, relationships with Jewish organizations are also at a very low level and exchanges of staff and members rarely take place. This applies also to the place of the Centre in the Jewish Welfare Board. Members of staff feel that the Centre occupies a marginal place in the Board's activities and that very little interest is shown by the Board's officials. This impression is due to a number of reasons ranging from the geographical distance between head office[18] and the Centre to the structure of the organization and its goals. To a certain extent, the Centre was regarded as a service quite distinct from other services provided by the Board, and hence as an independent unit inside the organization. The following letter sent by head office to participants demonstrates this point:

I would like to inform you that you will be receiving a grant to help you over the Passover and I hope that will be of some assistance. However, in view of the fact that we have opened a Day Centre in Marlsden with all the facilities that this has to offer, this grant will not be continued next year to people who are attending the Centre.

Until the appointment of an area team leader at head office to take charge of both the Centre and the Marlsden team, liaison between the Centre and the organization was irregular, loose and

unstructured. Board officials came every now and then to attend
staff meetings or to have a glance at the place, but this had no
effect on the running of the Centre or on policies pursued by its
staff. The only organizational enterprise the Centre was obliged to
take part in was the experimental merger with the Jewish Blind
Society Centre, and that was despite strong opposition from staff
as well as participants.

This particular decision gives us a perspective on the relationship
between the organization and the Centre. The Centre was a target
for attention and manipulation in so far as it could be used as a
resource for achieving certain organizational goals, but otherwise it
was neglected. Thus invitations to Board officials, asking for their
presence at activities and festivals held in the Centre, received no
response. Furthermore, as the Centre did not represent any attrac-
tion to potential donors, the Centre was kept from the attention of
benefactors. The Board's chief concern is that a successful image of
the Centre be maintained and disseminated amongst its sponsors
and that the place runs smoothly. As long as its growing attendance
causes no difficulties, the Board's involvement in the Centre is very
limited indeed.

However, intervention in the lives of individual participants was
often dictated by the social work done in the area by the Board's
staff. The nature of this work makes a substantial contribution to
the sequestration of the individual in a sanctuary, devoid of previous connections and affiliations. This results from the implementation of certain principles which underlie the ways social workers
approach their clients, conceive their problems, and deal with
them.

It has been suggested that a predominant aspect of society's attitude towards the elderly is the reduction of their personalities to
their material needs. However, the people who are in charge of
implementing this approach, social workers, are reluctant to view
their function merely in terms of the allocation of public resources
to meet these needs. This is unpalatable, it devalues their profession. Consequently, a subtle distinction between 'welfare officers'
and 'social workers' has been developed amongst members of the
Marlsden team. The crux of this differentiation is that 'welfare
officers', being traditionally the widely disliked agents of the notoriously patronizing, bureaucratic and unapproachable Jewish
Board of Guardians, evoked unpleasant connotations which might

impede relationships with the client. Thus, although the welfare side of the work was not belittled by the emphasis on the 'social work' function, it was nevertheless considered as merely an administrative facet of the job, requiring no special qualifications and by no means deserving the title of social work. Welfare is about 'material needs' while social work is about 'problems'. It was felt to be imperative that members of staff delineate the lines along which social work care to the client should be rendered, and hence a profile of the client's major problems was required.

When a positive response to a material application such as rehousing, financial aid, etc., is not forthcoming, social workers tend to find out the 'real' cause of distress by diverting their attention to another dimension of the client's life, which thereby becomes the cardinal target for care and concern. Thus dealing with a married couple who made numerous applications for accommodation, a social worker reported that: 'Both need to occupy themselves in a social contact and to get out in outings when these can be arranged. This seems to be a problem more overriding than that of accommodation.'

A widow who made a rehousing application was judged in this way:

> Mrs W. is a very depressed and bitter woman, she has had a most unhappy life. Now she tries to show that the whole problem is the accommodation and tries to repress all other problems. She threatened that she would commit suicide. All her aggression is towards herself. She seems to me to be a masochistic type of person.

This layman's use of psychological jargon is widespread and frequently employed to define and describe the clients' problems. Categorization such as 'paranoid', 'schizophrenic', 'sadistic', etc. serve one of two purposes. It may avert the possibility of being held responsible for the client's situation, for his problems are rooted in factors beyond their influence. Alternatively, it enables staff to prescribe the sort of treatment which is within their reach and entails no organizational difficulties in the form of trying to find resources and overcoming red tape. This 'treatment' is normally called 'a change of social environment', or, in more sophisticated terms, 'entering a therapeutic environment', i.e. the Centre.

In order to designate different clients to one place, designed to meet no specific problem, the social worker must eliminate a great deal of each client's special problems, background and idiosyncracies. This is done first and foremost by the development of a stereotyped conception of a client, based upon a series of premises concerning the essence of being an elderly hard-up Jewish Welfare Board applicant. There is the assumption that the typical client is an outcast from his family, and isolated from any social contact with friends and community. He is, therefore, completely dependent on the social worker and the liaison formed by him with welfare services. There is also the assumption that the typical client prefers Jewish care and hence has no viable alternative to his bond with the Jewish Welfare Board. These presuppositions, together with the view of the client as resisting change, but at the same time as being devoid of any constructive ideas and will of his own, easily manipulated and managed, complete the image of a client dependent on the social worker.

This concept is inculcated amongst social workers and supported by a philosophy on the advisable treatment. It includes certain unwritten rules guiding the expected attitude of the social worker. Usually these ideas are voiced in staff meetings and their main exponents are the senior social workers. One of the recurrent themes is that the social worker should forestall any possibility of the client's dependence on him. Thus if the client does cling to the social worker, it is despite the latter's intention. He is expected only to offer insight and advice, but not committed patronage. Another precept is that tampering with the client's personality should be strictly avoided. The social worker must direct his attention and efforts to the creation of a more comfortable environment for the client, but should refrain from any attempt to change him, to impose his values on him, or to pass moral judgment on his behaviour.

These rules of conduct are clearly not logical deductions from the conception of the client as a dependent, subject to manipulation. In fact, the rules refer to an ideological construction of the situation, whereas the assumptions stem from the daily encounters with applicants. This is a thematic incongruity which remains unnoticeable until a 'case' arises to expose it. Thus when a woman client offered an outstandingly systematic, sensible, and articulate interpretation of her plight, and asked the social worker in charge of her 'case' to refer it to the staff, a perplexed discussion ensued.

Here was a client asserting her personality and independence, in compliance with the rules, but in disagreement with the conception. Other instances of clients who refused to succumb to total dependence by rejecting assistance and opting to live under harsh conditions similarly baffled and intrigued their would-be benefactors.

In fact, measures are taken by social workers themselves to buttress the image of isolated, desperately needy people. Reports are full of vivid descriptions of social sequestration, desertion by families, hopelessness and helplessness. Although a great deal of this is undoubtedly factually true, there is a considerable bias towards selecting factors which validate the ruling conception.

A number of practical steps further established this view, especially with regard to the place of the family in the client's life. No attempts to contact children or other relatives were made, let alone attempts to verify the client's statements about his family. A suggestion that families be asked to contribute towards the cost of keeping one of their members in a Jewish Welfare Board old age home was rejected on the grounds that this would mean a reintroduction of the Jewish Board of Guardians' 'means test', and would involve undue interference in the relationship between the client and his family. The inevitable consequence was that the family was led to feel that its elderly member was being taken care of by the social worker, and that there was no call for them to share the responsibility for his welfare. This is a further, sometimes conclusive, step in the process of disengagement of the elderly person from his former social environment, and in his treatment as a separate entity.

This obliteration of the family from the scope of the social worker's activities is only one way in which aspects of the client's life with which the social worker prefers to have no dealings are excluded. To indicate some of these areas, I compare four day centre application forms, issued at different times. By following the change in emphasis, the omissions and additions, it will be possible to trace the process of diminishing concern with certain areas, and the disappearance of others.

Form 'A', the first to be introduced, was used from the inception of the Centre until 1973:

Form 'A'

JEWISH WELFARE BOARD   DAY CENTRE APPLICATION

1 Full Name   Case no.   Day Centre no.   Date of birth
   Address   Borough   Telephone no.
   Profession
2 Lives alone YES/NO
3 Family YES/NO
4 If yes, details:
5 Specific family support (visits)   Financial family support
6 Next of kin – Name   Tel. no.   In case of emergency
   neighbour or friend: Addresses
7 Home environment

State of health

 8 Diet (state)
 9 Emergency treatment
10 Physical limitations
11 Public transport YES/NO
12 Day Centre transport YES/NO Stairs YES/NO
13 Mental health history YES/NO. If yes, details
14 General medical information
15 GP's Name   Tel. no.
    Address

Domiciliary services

16 Home-help YES/NO – and when?
17 Voluntary worker, name   Tel. No.
    Address
18 Meals on Wheels YES/NO
19 District nurse YES/NO – and when?
20 Application for JWB flatlet YES/NO; Home YES/NO
    Category
21 Member of synagogue YES/NO, if yes, details
22 If no, what burial arrangements have been made
23 REMARKS

24 Retirement pension
25 Supplementary benefit
26 Sickness benefit
27 Rent
28 Savings

Full name of social worker   Date

This form was replaced by Form 'B', from which the following specifications were omitted:

Full name (only 'name' was asked for)/Day centre no.
Profession
Financial family support
Neighbour or friend to be contacted in case of emergency
Visits by family
Emergency transport
Day centre transport
General medical information
Voluntary worker visits
Membership of synagogue
Burial arrangements
Sickness benefits
Rent
Full name of social worker.

The information omitted refers mostly to the client's background, family connections, community affiliations and financial resources. All relate to the client's external life, and all are found to be immaterial to his Centre life. Nevertheless, some supplementary information was sought in Form 'B' about 'medication', 'days of attendance' and 'notes on personality', all pertinent to the client's participant role, and to the view that he is an independent, socially and psychologically self-sufficient individual.

Form 'C' carries the title of the Centre (instead of a general collective title referring to no specific centre in Forms 'A' and 'B') and includes the following specifications:

Date of first attendance

Name of the Centre

APPLICATION FORM

Name	Day Centre no.	Case no.	Date of birth
Address			Phone no.
Medical history			Diet:
GP			Phone:
Next of kin			Phone:
Reason for application			

Social worker   Date

No more enquiries about accommodation, family support, 'personality', welfare services, income, etc. Form 'D' which was a modification of 'C' does not include the administrative information relating to dates and names of social workers. These two last forms were devised during the fieldwork period.

Although medical information is vital in cases of emergency, social workers seem to be at odds with doctors' general assessments of their client and quite often dispute the validity of their judgment. It is rather common for a social worker to challenge a doctor's opinion of a patient's ability to cope with his situation. Such challenges invariably take the form of asserting the social worker's acquaintance with the case and his thorough knowledge of the client's attitudes and patterns of behaviour.

This dismissal of other professional involvement with the decisions concerning the client, together with the systematic obliteration of many aspects of the client's links with his surroundings, makes the social worker the sole liaison with the world and thus increases considerably the dependence of the client on his decisions. Furthermore, as this process means separation and disengagement from former ties and involvements, the client remains exposed to the influences and the forces of the situation created and manipulated for him by the social worker.

The result is that people's reluctance to accept charity is dissolved and their shame and 'integrity' is transformed into an excessive flow of applications for welfare assistance. This signifies the transformation from an external reference to an exploration of the options within the new boundaries set up by the social worker. The following report describes a social worker's first visit to a client:

> 'Mr J. was quite surprised at my visit and it later emerged that he was a very proud man – he stressed that he does not wish any charity. I explained to Mr J. that we were a welfare agency and that I had been asked to visit him by the hospital who were concerned about his welfare'.

Mr J. took advantage of this unexpected visit by asking for help in trying to sell his house. Then and ever since he has inundated the Board with various applications. This process recurs in most cases and it is quite evident that clients who become participants realize the potentialities of their new environment and adjust themselves to exploiting its resources. The Centre makes this environment tangible and defined not only by the daily contact with other applicants and the constant presence of social workers, but also by a process of gradual incorporation of outside services and activities into the Centre. This centralization makes the Centre a more total environment, comprehending a wide variety of aspects of the participants' lives. This totalization is in effect a delineation of boundaries emerging from the Centre itself and it consists of a number of elements.

TV licences, winter clothes, convalescence, telephone and electricity bills, etc. are all arranged and dealt with by the Centre's office. It is common for any query concerning eligibility for welfare entitlements, requests for legal advice, or complaints abut officialdom to be addressed to the office, and, indeed, these matters are often attended to. The grave accommodation situation of some participants is greatly alleviated by a liaison established for them by the office with landlords in the area, and with fellow participants who own property which could be sublet. The two notice boards covered with leaflets and notes on state benefits, community services and local events are an added dimension to the informative aspect of the Centre.

Information and advice, although facilitating communication with the outside world, cannot be a substitute for its resources. Such a replacement is partially achieved by the introduction into the Centre of several facilities which one would normally expect to seek in home surroundings. There is a special handicap bath for participants who are unable to use their own ordinary bathroom, and bathing itself is assisted, if necessary, by a member of staff. Participants may use the sewing machines and carpentry tools to do their own repairs, and the printing machine, as well as being used for Centre functions, serves the benevolent fund and even individual participants. Optical services, a barber (a participant), a beautician and a keep-fit instructor also contribute to the process of totalization.

Jumble sales and special sales (of kitchenware, clothes, etc.) are held frequently at the Centre, and most of them attract intensive interest from participants who otherwise could not afford to purchase some of the articles offered. The items are collected and sorted out by members of staff from local donors and participants. The stalls are manned by volunteers recruited amongst the participants under the supervision of staff. This method of recycling and redistributing participants' resources produces a certain degree of self-sufficiency and independence of the outside world, which is one of the constituents of the autonomous isolated character of the Centre.

This aspect is accentuated by a growing demand by participants to expand the Centre's operation to Saturdays and late evenings. The closing of the premises on certain holidays caused a great deal of grievance, and the refusal of staff to comply with the demand to prolong the opening hours was responsible for several altercations and outbursts. When the new supervisor took office he tried to use the demand for extended activities to achieve full employment of his staff, in order to curb the leakage of resources from the Centre into the constituency of the Marlsden team and its leader, who was the supervisor's superior.

Participants were ready to do their share in such an expansion of the Centre's activities. Handicapped participants were encouraged to ask for family attendance in the Centre, especially by wives who stayed at home whilst their husbands spent the day at the Centre. Sunday activities were well attended by participants and special events held in the evenings proved to be indisputable successes.

The persistence and relish expressed by participants in fuelling the process of totalization is closely linked with their conception of the significance of the Centre in their lives. This is by no means a unanimous approach, nor is it a clear, articulate system of ideas and concepts. It is rather a collection of attitudes and behaviour emerging from occasional conversations and everyday situations, and deriving from the nature of the care system (see 'The idea of care'). Nevertheless, some predominant characteristics of the ways participants see their relationship with the Centre may be sorted out with reference to three issues referred to and discussed by participants – (a) what the Centre is not; (b) the uniqueness of relationships in the Centre; (c) the place of the Centre in the overall organization of its participants' lives.

Any attempt made in discussion groups or during other activities to broach the subject of the definition of the Centre, invariably provoked confusion and indecision. People constantly failed to suggest an acceptable label for the establishment. Usually general agreement prevailed as to the non-characteristics of the Centre. Thus, the Centre is by no means only a luncheon club, nor is it merely a recreation centre. It is neither a voluntary friendship club nor a compulsory environment, such as a workhouse. These institutions, standing at either end of the authority scale, were consistently eliminated from a comparison, the former because of its uncommitted, limited purpose membership, the latter in response to direct or indirect acquaintance with the notoriously dehumanizing, strict regime in these institutions.

There is also agreement on the admissibility of candidates into the Centre. People who come to the Centre to pursue only unsociable interests, such as enjoying a cheap meal, and having their own clothes repaired, were unwanted, and disturbing elements. Another criterion is the applicant's economic position. Attendance in the absence of financial hardship, although obviously motivated by other difficulties, is often frowned upon, and considered an abuse of the Centre's fundamental mission, which is catering for the poor. Thus it is not uncommon to see participants deliberately belittling their income and other resources to persuade their fellow members that their claim to be recognized and accepted in the Centre is fully justified from an economic point of view.

Given sociability and poverty, one is acceptable. Participants agree that the Centre is a heterogeneous environment, capable of, and designed to, absorb and welcome applicants who face some sort of difficulty, regardless of age, mental state or physical condition. An attempt to circulate a petition concerning the plight of old age pensioners was aborted by the committee on the grounds that

'this is not a Centre only for old people and it should not be identified as such'. Likewise, criticism of participants who seemed to
enjoy good health were regarded as 'unfair' because 'there are
.many other reasons apart from disablement why people should
attend the Centre'.

The heterogeneity of the Centre is one basis for the prevailing
feeling of participants that it is a unique environment, quite different from other, superficially comparable establishments. The terminology used is illuminating. Participants often talk of each other as
'brothers and sisters' or even 'closer than family'. A participant
who wanted to phrase the difference in feeling between the Centre
and the Fridays at the Jewish Blind Society Centre compared the
former to a 'mother's home' whereas the latter was depicted as a
'step-mother's home'. This analogy to a 'home' was seconded and
elaborated on by many other participants who reiterated their view
of the Centre as the only significant facet of their existence. Some
went even further, saying that entering the Centre was a life-giving
transformation for them.

Participants see the Centre as an arena where one can start a
whole new range of relationships and transform one's self-image.
A few even say that 'in the Centre you are just yourself', meaning
that one can act out all the roles to which one used to aspire. One
can play the role of a manager, an artist, a workingclass politician,
etc. without the threat of being ridiculed or dismissed as 'being out
of your mind'. Jonathan, one of the leading participants, recalled a
folk tale from his Polish *shtetel*:

> 'In our *shtetel* there used to be a broad log of wood in the middle
> of the marketplace. Every midnight the souls of the dead
> gathered around it and each of them behaved and talked the way
> he wanted to be in his real life.
> The shoemaker became the warden of the synagogue, the
> water-drawer was the rabbi, and the poor tailor sat in the
> Mayor's chair. And they were all satisfied and happy.'

The social mechanism behind this conception of the Centre can
be left for later discussion, but the conception itself is significant
for the understanding of the relationship between the Centre world
and the outside. Whereas the non-Centre world contains rejection,
disintegration, sequestration and alienation, the fraternal environment created in the Centre offers just the opposite. There are no

insuperable internal barriers between participants. The Centre is perceived as a communication system through which almost any message can be conveyed and fed back. This is based on the realization that participants are isolated from the outside world but remain free to regulate their participation as they like. There is therefore no way of imposing outside values on the other participants.

The borderline separating the two worlds is maintained. The Centre is viewed as an alternative reality, and any interpenetration with the outside world is regarded as undesirable, and contaminating. Thus a participant who was 'caught' in the local park chatting to non-participants about the Centre was told off by fellow members, who warned him not to involve the Centre in his 'private life'. Participants who seemed to establish fairly close friendships in the Centre rarely extended their relationships outside, and this despite consistent encouragement to do so from staff. The very few occasions when meetings took place outside were either initiated and organized by the Centre (outings), or derived directly from the activities in the Centre (rehearsals for a concert).

This strict demarcation of the Centre from other environments is probably the most significant characteristic of the Centre's boundaries. Community alienation, organizational structure and social workers' policies are all involved in the creation of a social environment highly distinct from its surroundings. What are the relationships between this isolated haven and the nature of the limbo state?

None of the incongruities of the limbo state are solved or mitigated by the mere setting of the Centre. Society's attitude towards the elderly remains unchanged and the processes of personal deterioration and disintegration continue. Nevertheless, the sharp distinction between the Centre and its outside environment may provide a new basis for the development of attitudes and conceptions which could be used as responses to these problems. This is not to say that different circumstances would not produce similar reactions, but apparently there is a direct correlation between the structure of the Centre as described in this chapter and the management of the limbo predicament.

The Centre is in fact an autonomous, self-contained and self-sufficient unit, and it is highly separated from the influences, forces and constraints of the social environment of pre-Centre existence.

It is a social enclave, but not in the sense that no social life exists there; on the contrary, it is difficult to envisage a more hectic, turbulent environment. However, it is an enclave in so far as definite and special rules, regulations, norms and expectations are imposed on the participants. The amount of freedom to choose, and opportunities for manipulation, are exceptional, and are not comparable to what other elderly people often experience in regimented institutions, or under the control of a resentful family, or whilst leading a lonely housebound life. Few demands are made of participants, and freedom to handle the balance between Centre attendance and outside life is complete. In this respect the Centre is a flexible, undemanding environment which enables people to make their own decisions on how to conduct their lives whilst offering them a multitude of facilities.

It is in the opportunities offered for decision-making that life in the Centre contrasts with the limbo state. In the limbo state, the power to influence one's own fate is considerably curtailed, whereas in the Centre every opportunity is given to people to mould their relationships and behaviour, within the boundaries of the setting.

The fact that socially the Centre is segregated from other environments circumscribes the permeation of the attitudes and values engendering the limbo state to a minimum. Should a participant leave the Centre, even temporarily, a fresh confrontation with the limbo state is inevitable, although the effect of participation might alleviate it. Nevertheless, so long as attendance is maintained, the Centre provides a safe harbour for not only ephemeral escape and refuge, but even for dealing with the fundamental predicaments of the limbo state.

As the main incongruities of the limbo state are encapsulated in the contradictory perception of time experienced by the elderly, an attempt will be made to follow the reactions developed to it in the Centre through the handling of the ingredients of time by the participants. The leading question to be put is 'what are the ways employed by participants to resolve the contradiction between static social time and the degeneration which characterizes personal time?' A sociological treatment of this question will be possible only after an examination of the nature of the Centre as a social environment in contrast to the outside world. The relationship between the two underpins the discussion of participants' time perspectives.

3   Reordering time

Turning now to the participants' perspectives on the Centre, and its relationship with its environment, their sense of time requires special consideration. It is of crucial importance, yet in no way obvious. People rarely speak of 'time', and then only in relation to situations outside the Centre; and particularly with respect to 'passing time'. People say, 'I went to the cinema to kill a couple of hours', or, 'I am going to my club just to pass the time', almost as though time does not exist in the Centre itself, but is capable of being a nuisance outside. Though it is both elaborate and significant, their concept of time must be sought obliquely.

It will be recalled that the limbo state encapsulates three discrepant experiences of time. (a) The past, the life history of the individual, loses its meaning. (b) The official solution to their plight involves seclusion, often institutionalization, and, effectively, the freezing of their social condition. (c) This is incongruous with the actual experience of accelerating deterioration, and the consciousness of death, in which time is eliminated. Dealing with the limbo state means resolving these conflicts, and each facet is dealt with here in turn.

Revising the past

Initial encounters with the Centre tend to be baffling. As a trainee social worker commented on her first day in the Centre: 'these people have obviously had a rich and interesting past, and yet it seems as if they all live in the present, engrossed with their day-to-day lives.' This dissociation from the past was so marked that social workers used it as a yardstick to assess the progress of a participant in integrating himself into the Centre. Thus, a woman who rejected the idea of attending the Centre was found to be in a state of 'depression, withdrawal, occasional tearfulness - dwells on past tragedies'. Another newcomer who did not show a 'satis-factory adjustment' was described as 'obsessed with her memories – drifts in and out of Centre'. Many other outsiders were also struck by the apparent reluctance of participants to engage in any activity relating to their pre-Centre existence. A representative of a community organization who sought the participants' assistance in compiling historical material on Marlsden received no significant response from most of the participants, who seemed to be uninterested and even deliberately obstructive. On another occasion a talk was given on the East End at the turn of the century – the cradle of the majority of the participants. This time a substan-tial group of members actively opposed the event, arranging enter-tainments on the upper floor simultaneously with the speaker's appearance in the dining room. The upper hall was an entirely new arena for afternoon activities, and it was used on that occasion in order to draw attention from, and, perhaps, disrupt the talk.

During a home visit to one of the participants I indirectly pro-voked a quarrel between the husband and his wife – both partici-pants. The man tried to tell me some of his adventures as a stow-away en route to America. His wife interrupted: 'don't dramatize, it is all in the past and therefore not interesting; in any case we are not sure it really happened.' There was a loud altercation when the man tried to describe his skirmishes with anti-Semitic thugs in the area.

A similar reaction, though less personal, was directed at a local councillor who came to the Centre to talk about problems in the educational system. After a few minutes of polite attention he was impatiently interrupted and asked to change the subject as 'we are not children or parents any more and our education is in the past – we don't want to hear about it'. Some of the audience left the room.

New participants usually do try to reflect upon their past, but are confronted by an apathetic reaction from the veterans, some-times accompanied by explanatory remarks such as 'we are here to forget our past not to brood upon it; the Centre is for people who want to forget their troubles' (see 'Initiation'). This sense of the meaninglessness of trying to relive the past was conveyed in a form of a short story by one of the participants, published in *News and Views*.

This is a story of an alcoholic ex-film actor, named Ralph, who goes to see one of his old performances and gets involved in a brawl with a spectator over the quality of his acting and, consequently, is taken to the police station. The police officer, after hearing what happened, gives his advice: 'There is no use living in the past.' 'Ralph nodded and was reminded of the bump on his head (a result of the brawl). The sergeant looked sympathetically at Ralph who at that moment left like a complete fool.'

The realization that the past, even a glamorized one, is irredeemable and irreversible was emphatically reiterated by participants, and they firmly rejected attempts by staff to get them to reflect on it. A discussion group on the subject, 'what would you do if you could relive your life?' attracted nobody, until the staff actively persuaded people to attend. The discussion then took the form of a semantic debate on the validity of the use of the conditional term, 'if'. Two speakers argued that as the past could not have been changed anyway, the topic was futile and meaningless. The debate was continually interrupted – deviations from the subject, cross talk, private conversations and jokes filled most of the time, until the chairman abandoned his efforts, and the group was dispersed.

Joking was a common way of dealing with past experiences. Thus a woman participant who insisted on giving a full account of her life in the East End, in a discussion group, was treated as a joke-teller. Every event she described provoked laughter and a cheer. It was as if life in the East End was so remote as to be absurd.

Nevertheless, there are times when the mask of indifference is removed and participants give way to uncontrollable nostalgia. Such an incident occurred when a group of outside entertainers appeared at the Centre for a Chanukah party. They sang their usual repertoire of popular songs from the 1920s and 1930s, and, as they wanted to please their audience, ended the show with 'A Yiddisha Mama'. This triggered off an immediate and unexpected outburst of sobbing and emotion, which turned to dismay and fury. A few participants loudly abused the performers for introducing unsuitable entertainment, 'pouring salt on our wounds and opening old scars'. Having comforted each other, the participants demanded a return to the frivolities of musical and cabaret songs. The incident was not mentioned again in the Centre.

Such incidents reveal that the past is, indeed, indelible, and although no effort is spared to erase substantial parts of it, its impact on the Centre is still considerable. In fact, a more careful and thorough examination of references to the past reveals that there is some consistency in the way participants review and edit their biographies.

Three major techniques are used. The first is complete erasure, the second renunciation, and the third is to cherish, sometimes glorify nostalgically, events. The manifestation of these attitudes can be intermittently detected in the way life histories are presented in the Centre. There are significant differences between various participants' versions of their biographies, but certain common denominators do prevail. I shall outline the phases of the life cycles and locate the operation of the three monitors.

Parents were depicted with a compound of respect, shame and disapproval. The way participants were brought up in the East End at the turn of the century was viewed as entirely misplaced and inadequate. Being sent to religious schools, goaded to conform to a strict orthodox way of life, not being given the opportunity to assi-milate English culture, were all points of criticism. Acrimony and regret dominated participants' attitudes towards their parents. This was fused with an unfavourable image of their parents' generation as narrow-minded, unreasonable and rigidly religious, failing to integrate to its social environment and to find an honourable, respectable form of living.

The picture of domestic life was even gloomier. Hardworking, constantly exhausted mothers were burdened with a bunch of untidy, unclean, screaming children. Fathers were short-tempered, demanding, precariously employed and invariably experienced dif-ficulty in sustaining the family. Housing was cramped and squalid and the burden of looking after oneself came early, fourteen- to fifteen-year-old members of the family having to go to work. It was by no means conceived of as a childhood of stability, security and good prospects, and an implicit condemnation of those held res-ponsible limited any reference to it.

Community life on the other hand was viewed in a much more nostalgic light. Friendship and neighbourliness were the main features of life in that close-knit small Jewish surrounding. This was a period of gaiety, outdoor enjoyments such as dances, parties and late night outings, sustained by inexhaustible vigour and vita-lity. People used to talk to one another, to offer help and to show genuine concern and interest. This was, of course, contrasted to the disregard and alienation which characterized modern society.

These descriptions of conviviality and fraternity applied to the phase of young adulthood until marriage, after which a significant gap was noticed. Participants rarely talked about their married life, the way they brought up their children, and particularly their occupations and socio-economic positions. Thus a man who was a leading tailor did mention this fact to me, but refrained from discussing it openly with other participants (a great number of them former tailors too, though less successful). Another participant, who was a well-to-do costermonger, also scarcely spoke about his trade in the market, although he was willing enough to discuss the most intimate personal problems. A participant who had written and published a few short stories and was working on his autobiography never mentioned this fact to fellow participants or to staff and visitors.

This tendency to erase occupational histories came out in a discussion group when those present were asked to speak freely about their lives. There was firm opposition to any reference to 'later life', and participants who did not comply were instantly called to order. One person said: 'Since I was seventeen years old I started to think for myself and what I did with my bloody life is my own business.'

Newcomers to the Centre who tried to talk about this aspect of their lives were often taken aback by the inattention and indifference shown by their listeners. Usually the message got across quickly, and they responded by joining the 'pastless' others. The rule applies not only to the discussion of occupations but also hobbies, love affairs, communal activities and voluntary work.

Social workers are amazed at the speedy recovery participants in the Centre make from a state of grief and bereavement to a 'normal', complaisant attitude towards the loss of a spouse. Sometimes it was only a matter of days between the arrival of a shattered and depressed newcomer at the Centre and the emergence of a present-oriented participant, enjoying the Centre atmosphere. When participants do mention a deceased spouse it is usually with reference to their early lives together, and very rarely to more recent events.

Men depicted their late wives as loving and caring, while women participants tended to give a less idealistic account of their family relationship. Some would even admit that the marriage was forced upon them, and that they are not sure what love means, as it never entered their feelings towards their husbands. Both widows and widowers – though particularly widowers – expressed a desire to be rid of those relics which every now and again recalled an irrecoverable past.

Children, however, did not fit into this nostalgic vision. The attitude towards them was motivated by the awareness of their alienation and desertion, causing a strong element of voluntary disengagement on the part of the parents. Participants openly discussed their bitter disillusionment and anger at their children's behaviour towards them, ànd, often expressed determination not to let the relationship disturb their lives any more. In consequence an attitude of renunciation of children developed in the Centre. Participants publicly regretted the fact that they had brought children into the world and said that if they were to live their lives over again they would not repeat this grave mistake. Stories circulated by participants about their own bitter disenchantment with their children served to corroborate and intensify this view.

On *seder* night (Passover eve) the Centre was crammed with participants who preferred to celebrate in the company of their fellow participants rather than to join their families. Some of those present chose to emphasize that although their families had invited them home they had made it clear that their loyalties and sympathies rested with their fellow participants, and, therefore, had opted for the Centre. The fact that the *seder* is usually a major annual occasion for family gatherings was recognized, however, and a number of participants remarked on the anomaly of having to resort to a completely inadequate, 'pathetic' substitute.

One woman had expected to receive an invitation to the *seder* at her son's home, but it did not materialize. On the night of the *seder* she was picked up by her son and left at the doors of the Centre while he drove away to his home. She could not accept the rebuff and maintained that she would be collected by her son to celebrate the festival with her grandchildren. The son never came and the bewildered mother had to be comforted by more experienced parents, who explained to her their views on the meaninglessness of the relationship between the generations.

The very common practice amongst old people of exchanging family photographs and enjoying mutual adoration of the children and grandchildren (Johnson, 1971, p.77) rarely took place in the Centre. 'Paper children' – as some participants preferred to call such pictures – were produced mostly if the subjects were living abroad, and so no excuse for their remoteness would have to be contrived by the parents. People were, indeed, interested in photographs, but mostly of themselves either as youngsters or as participants at present. One of the activities which took place before fieldwork started, but which left a considerable impact on the participants' memories, was a photographic contest, described by a member of staff as follows:

> 'A highly successful photo quiz was organized, each member having produced anonymously a photograph of himself as a youngster or young adult, the aim being for the other members to guess who was who. This quiz provoked a great deal of conversation and interest between the members who became happily reminiscent.'

The fun of putting together the remote past and present by comparing youthful and old physical appearance seems to indicate that there was some desire amongst participants to relate to their past and to maintain a certain sense of continuity interlinking their life-history. Indeed, excursions into the past were occasionally made in the Centre, but they were carefully selected and included only those elements which seem to suggest no strains, and which did not indicate differences between participants. In effect they help to produce a shared pattern of time, divorced from personal careers and quirks, and stripped of all the socially conceived injustices which have brought about the limbo state. As will become clear, this selective past resembles the notion of the present moulded in the Centre.

The parts of the past recalled readily and unapologetically concerned situations of seeming social equality. Thus participation in the big East End demonstrations in the 1930s against the Fascist movement was proudly recalled, and these stories encouraged participants to recall their youthful political affiliations, with their associations of comradeship and fraternity. Similarly, war-time and army service were viewed as the heyday of sharing, joint effort and unconditional friendship. They ignored its rigid hierarchy when discussing the army, and similarly stressed equality and ignored hierarchy in discussing hospitals.

Most participants have been hospitalized more than once and they possess an extensive experience of such establishments. Reminiscences of hospital include praise for the medical staff, but emphasize the cordial relationship, and the lack of social barriers, between the patients. A number of participants commented in terms usually restricted to the Centre reality. Thus several said, 'I became a new person there', or 'They gave me a new life.'

While participants who were acquainted with each other in their pre-Centre life normally make no mention of this fact, and sometimes relate to each other as if they have first met in the Centre, being in the same hospital ward is an accepted ground for a continuous relationship. Participants treat that shared experience on the same level as they conceive their co-existence in the Centre and the time lapse separating these two phases in their lives seems to be irrelevant.

Friendship clubs, pubs and other informal communities are also recalled by participants. A man of over seventy used to claim active membership of twenty-two different clubs and societies. A friend in the Centre said he was 'one who will never grow old, simply because he does not live in the past'. He chose to separate from his wife, had no contact whatsoever with his only daughter and moved to an isolated, self-contained bedsitter where he lived on his own. In this complete detachment from the past, the only continuity was his attendance at clubs.

The life review of participants is far more than a psychological self-reflection (Butler, 1964), it is a social revision of past experiences, an adaptation to the Centre reality. Three different techniques of elimination are used – obliteration, renunciation and equalization. One eliminates elements in one's life which are contradictory and disruptive to the construction of a new relationship between participants. Thus, inequality and differences are obliterated. Family relationships, especially those with children, were also renounced, but the very strength of the renunciation indicates the tensions and deep feelings still aroused by these relationships.

The common thread linking East End political demonstrations, army service, war-time life, hospitals and social clubs links them in turn to the social reality created in the Centre. This issue will be discussed later, but some of the critical features of these experiences may be briefly indicated. They are all periods when life was apparently static, and these experiences were not stages in individual careers. Above all, they involved groups with specific values not shared outside.

References to countries of origin, holidays abroad, or to foreign places in general were scarce: always with the exception of Israel. They talked of visits to Israel, of service there in the British army, of children living there and of voluntary Zionist work. They expressed not only attachment but a feeling of belonging there. Participants could be very critical of particular Israeli policies, or of aspects of life there, but their basic feeling was one of loyalty and patriotism. They realized that their chances of going to Israel, even on a visit, were slim. One participant remarked, 'They don't want and they don't need people like us, old and handicapped.' Yet there was this overriding feeling that their Israel, an unattainable, unreal reality, was the only alternative reality to that provided by the Centre. All other possibilities were persistently and decisively rejected.

Alternative realities

The tantalizing, sometimes ominous, existence of alternatives demand a persistent, endless effort to invalidate, cognitively to obliterate them. There are two types of such alternatives. The first are not necessarily exclusive of attendance at the Centre, such as religion and family, while the second involve alternative environments superseding the Centre. Two different, although complementary, ways of confronting alternative realities were employed by participants. The first, which following Berger and Luckmann (1966, p.130) might be called 'annihilation', involves devaluing their significance. The second, however, aims at forestalling them. What makes these two strategies viable is their common foundation in an overall conception of relations between events, that has been developed and elaborated in the Centre. This is fundamentally a fatalistic view based on the premise that the course of events is beyond human control and, therefore, a link between cause and effect is due to sheer luck or is completely coincidental. I shall now discuss the way in which this fatalistic conception is constituted, and its implications for the invalidation of alternative realities.

Participants explicitly described themselves on numerous occasions as 'fatalists', meaning that they were at the mercy of circumstance and the deeds of other people. The factor of 'luck' or 'fate' is invoked as a reluctant admission that there might be some external power determining the flow of events. This agent is referred to by participants exclusively in secular terms, and it seems that its dubious, undefined existence serves merely to impart some coherence to the anarchic connection between cause and effect.

One recurrent element underlining the conception is the belief that nothing is really in a process of change and progression. Thus the argument that children's lives are no different to the lives of their parents, and that society's attitude towards the elderly is very much the same as it always has been, are pressed to the conclusion that as events are beyond one's control and are not likely to get worse or better, the right approach to life is one of 'wait and see' – an attitude ruling out any intentional interference, and adapted to any circumstances, covering a range from family situations to political and social viewpoints. Some of its main manifestations will be described here, although a more comprehensive discussion will be found later, in the analysis of the care system.

Success or failure in marriage is a matter of mere 'luck'. As one of the participants said: 'It is like a gamble and you have got to take your chance.' The spouses' contribution to the marriage is dismissed as immaterial to the end result, and so is the way children are brought up. They recognize no correlation between what was invested in the child – both financially and emotionally – and the attention and support given by him to his parents. Thus the expectation of reciprocity is replaced by a stress on the haphazard and unpredictable.

The view that life is a gamble[1] has a special bearing where health and illness are concerned. Suggestions that certain ailments could be reasonably treated and even that a complete recovery might be effected were dismissed casually as inapplicable to the present and dubious in the future. Mistrust of doctors was prevalent, and stories concerning medical errors, contradictory treatments, disagreements within the medical profession, disregard and negligence were constantly circulated. Denying the possibility of recovery involved challenging the expertise of professionals. Thus new discoveries concerning the nature and causes of multiple sclerosis were judged to be premature and speculative by participants who suffered from this disease. The same people treated with disbelief the claims of a multiple sclerosis patient that somehow, by using a carefully balanced diet, he had managed to cure himself of the disease.

As neither personal experience nor professional advice are considered of any avail, the predominant view that the prognosis is uncertain remains unchallenged. Yet participants usually refer to their medical condition as if it was static. No cure is to be expected, but deterioration is unlikely. Thus people with terminal diseases speak freely of their present hardships, but rarely contemplate a possible worsening in their condition. The implicit feeling is that the Centre is a sanctuary, impervious to the ordinary processes of change dominating the 'normal' course of events in the outside world. Such an attitude was expressed by a participant who knew that his condition was incurable, and aware of the inevitable end. 'I am living from one moment to another and I am what I am and that's all there is to it.' This distils the conception of time created in the Centre, and it applies to the state of health as well as to other aspects of life.

Retirement is also a situation beyond planning. In a discussion held on this subject participants agreed unanimously that as no one could predict the future, there is not much point in trying to plan. There was agreement that for most of them retirement had marked a change for the worse, but nobody would concede that this could have been averted had a planned retirement been designed.

The shame associated with dependence on the Jewish Welfare Board is also mitigated by the inevitability of the dependence. Participants blame their social position on forces beyond their control, and just as 'luck' brought them to the Centre, another unpredictable event might terminate the Centre phase in their lives. Thus participants who were asked about their Centre arrangements for a few weeks or even days ahead often shrugged off the query. They did not know what the future had in store for them. Many undertakings were preceded by the remark 'If I am still here' and a failure to meet an obligation was not regarded as a breach of the expectations.

There is an evident logical contradiction between the way participants refer to the Centre as an unchangeable environment and their fatalistic approach to the prospect of having to leave it. For if change has been obliterated, what are the sources of the risks of being forced to quit? The contradiction is between their resignation before fate and the view of the Centre as an isolated haven segregated from the effect of outside rules.

As no prediction is applicable to the Centre reality, the concept of progress or even a teleological process is of no significance to participants. Events in the Centre certainly do not follow one another in a linear way, nor do they take an orderly, cyclical form. In fact, they tend to be encapsulated aggregates composed of an unrelated, separate series of connected activities. This concept will be enlarged on later, but it would be appropriate to stress here that as there is no teleological link between events, planning is meaningless.

Perhaps the best expression of this philosophy was given by a participant who covered bottles with mosaic. To the question as to what he intended to do after he would finish coating one bottle, he replied, 'I will probably make another one and then another and so on, no end.' He did not express any desire to improve on his work, to excel by making more bottles than other participants, or to be rewarded either materially or socially.

Changes in the outside world do, however, call for an interpretation, and it is then that participants talk in terms of 'luck', 'fate', etc. Thus differences between rich and poor, between social classes, between the healthy and the sick, and transformations from one extreme to another, are all put down to the dicey operation of chance.

Even adherence to religious practice is attributed to circumstances, such as having a religious wife, or being subject to a father's persuasion and social pressures. Only one of the participants would confess that certain religious phases in his past had been due to his own choice and conviction. The denial of free will was nicely illustrated in the argument advanced by a participant to deny any possibility of his committing a sin. According to him, as the concept of sin contained the element of intention, he could not be regarded as a sinner since he had never chosen deliberately to defy God, and that if he did trespass it was accidental and, therefore, was not culpable.

This denial of any deliberate religious affiliation is part and parcel of the overall attitude in the Centre towards any belief in the supernatural, and particularly towards the Jewish religion as an alternative reality. Most of the participants had been acquainted in their childhood and young adulthood with strict observance of the Jewish faith and at present they have daily encounters with members of some of the most orthodox sects in Judaism. The British centre of the Lubavitz Hassidic sect – a world-wide movement for the return to practising Judaism – is nearby. Occasional encounters with its missionary representatives are unavoidable.

This rejection of religion involves, first, disenchantment with religious institutions and the conceived religious way of life, and second, a denial of fundamental religious notions such as the idea of Divine Providence, the after-life, and the connection of evil and good with reward and punishment. All represent an alternative reality based upon an entirely different idea of time, rooted in the past and stretching into the future.

The very mention of religion causes loud protests, and any proposed discussion associated with the subject is invariably strongly opposed. Participants are adamant in their insistence that religion be excluded from the Centre world. Members of staff, being well aware of this taboo, are very cautious about broaching any related topic. On the very rare occasion when such issues are not brushed aside, participants unanimously deny the validity of religious belief and reject religious practice. A discussion group on the supernatural, reluctantly attended at the Jewish Blind Society Centre, took the form of arguments completely denying super-natural phenomena. Participants soon decided that as there was no noticeable opposition to their line the topic was exhausted, and a new subject was brought up. A religious but inexperienced social worker managed to attract leading participants to a series of discussions on religion, but only because they wanted to help him in his initial steps in the Centre, by attending his activities. Most of the information on the attitude towards religion is, therefore, extracted from these meetings.

A great number of participants are members of synagogues, as this is the only way to ensure Jewish burial arrangements. As actual attendance at the synagogue is negligible, the membership fees required by the synagogue administration seem to be exorbitant and unfair, particularly in view of the subscribers' economic hard-ships. The fact that no concessions are made on this ground adds to the feeling that, as one of the participants once put it, 'they are all extortionists, money-mad'. Stories about ill-treatment are retailed with fury in the Centre. One participant claimed that he was virtually expelled from a synagogue on the Day of Atonement as a non-member of the congregation. Another described how he was snubbed by the warden of his synagogue because he had been in arrears with his bills. One experience particularly incensed the par-ticipants. It was the allegation of a man confined to a wheelchair that he was refused admission to his own synagogue on a Saturday, not because there were no adequate facilities to accommodate him, but because the Rabbi defined the wheelchair as a vehicle breaching the law against using transport on the Sabbath.

Participants used these stories to attack a Lubavitz Rabbi who came to the Centre three times of his own accord, and eventually was asked not to bother to come again. Despite his articulate and apologetic defence, his arguments remained unacceptable. Indeed, it triggered off another flow of accusations, about exorbitant food prices incurred by Kashruth[2] regulations, and the strictness and over-payment of the Shomers.[3] The Rabbi's attempt to produce an explanation based on religious lore was dismissed by the participants as irrelevant, for it did not take into account humane considerations which should have received absolute priority.[4] A number of people acrimoniously remarked on what seemed to them to be the discriminating attitude of institutional Judaism towards the poor and the socially deprived. They claimed that well-to-do Jews disregard the plight of their less fortunate brethren.

This critique of religious people recurs in various forms, and sometimes leads to blunt or even abusive expressions. The most common accusation is of hypocrisy and double standards. Some participants pursued this line of argument to its logical conclusions and formulated the syllogism that if religion is what people practise and observe, and if this practice yields unfavourable consequences, then religion as a whole is an evil practice.

Some participants went further, criticizing fundamental Jewish beliefs. The first notion to be seriously questioned was the existence of God. Roughly, the main line of argument was as follows: if there is a God, He must be just, and as there is no justice in this world, there is no God. Counter arguments presented by the orthodox social worker were rejected as 'philosophical'. Another line of argument had a similar practical conclusion. Even if God does exist He is either ruthless or not concerned with this world. In either case He is not worth worshipping. As one of the participants put it, 'If this is God I don't want anything to do with Him.' The major substantiation of this argument, regularly cited, was the Nazi holocaust, taken as evidence either of the non-existence of God, or of His ruthlessness. It was invariably the ultimate argument in such discussions and whenever the subject was broached it produced highly emotive outbursts, even crying and sobbing. Utterances such as 'There *was* a God' and 'God is dead' were typical.

Their conclusion applied far beyond the boundaries of Judaism. Participants would not accept any suggestion that there is another form of meaningful life in the time-bounded outside world. Two incidents demonstrate this point.

Sam did not involve himself with many other participants and chose to spend most of the day idling in an armchair, or chatting to a very select group of friends. He was separated from his wife. He had two children, whom he renounced and, not having seen them for twenty years, they played no role in his present life. His accommodation was a bedsitter with no cooking facilities or private sanitation. A stroke which he had suffered a few years ago erased, according to him, most of his past memories and apart from the fact that he had been in the leather trade, very little was known about his life history.

Had it not been for one aspect of Sam's life he could have been featured as the epitome of the Centre virtues. This aspect was his preoccupation with spiritualism. Sam was in his time a leading member of the Jewish spiritualist society. He had chaired his own seance circle, met with the most prominent figures in the field and gained a versatile and rich experience in the field. All this was completely ignored by his fellow participants despite Sam's attempts to win their attention and interest. He advocated a coherent theory concerning the ascent of the soul to other levels of existence and its journey to the complex after-life. One might have thought that such ideas would appeal to people on the verge of death, but the fact was that Sam found no audience in the Centre for his teachings. None of the other participants paid heed to his spiritualistic talk, although they were quite willing to listen to him speaking on other subjects.

However, a few women participants made an approach to Sam in an attempt to induce him to elaborate on his favourite subject in a special discussion group. Participants were assembled and Sam was called downstairs. As soon as he started it was evident that the things he intended to say were well prepared and that Sam was delighted to have been given the opportunity to speak. Nevertheless, he remained unheard. A massive opposition to the talk was immediately formed and Sam was prevented from continuing. Despite repeated requests to stay and contribute to another discussion, he left the room in a rage.

Another incident when participants almost exerted physical force to ostracize a speaker on the supernatural occurred when a faith-healer came to speak about his beliefs and to demonstrate his powers. A man who had appeared a few weeks earlier as a musical entertainer in a show organized for the participants, offered his services in his other capacity, and was invited by a member of staff to demonstrate them. Usually external speakers are treated in the Centre with tolerance and attention. Even if there is a fundamental disagreement with the line of argument taken by the speaker, he is patiently listened to and comments and questions are raised politely and in an orderly way. In the event of an accidental breach of these norms by an over-excited or peevish participant, he is quickly called to order. This pattern also prevailed at the beginning of the faith-healer's talk.

He spoke about the death of his wife and the impact of the bereavement on his life, and this won him sympathetic attention from his audience. He went on to relate his experience in contacting the dead, and here there was a discernible disquiet among participants. When he started describing experiments in table levitation and seances an upsurge of jeers and deliberate interruptions made the continuation of the talk virtually impossible. People began to exchange jokes and to insult him – e.g. 'You'd better heal yourself first from your stupidity.' There was nobody to control the situation, and the uproar grew. The astounded faith-healer, who was about to put on his gown to start practising, had hurriedly to collect his articles and, having sworn not to visit the Centre again, walked out, frightened and shattered.

The outrage was not reflected in further discussions and meetings and only two notable references were made to me. The first was a demand to erase the recording of the talk from my machine, since 'That man is living in a world of charade; there is no truth in what he was saying and his lies should not be allowed even to remain on tape.' The second reference was a remark made confidentially to me, that in future such talks should be aborted before they start as 'we are all old people and it is cruel to delude us with such nonsense'.

This contrived obliteration of religion and the whole field of alternative, unearthly realities applies also to the very mundane arena of political affairs. Participants explicitly and firmly object to any introduction of political subjects into discussion groups, and politics are mentioned in the same breath with religion as issues alien to the Centre atmosphere. National and international affairs are rarely discussed, and newspapers are brought to the Centre (mainly the *Daily Mirror* and the *Sun*) only for their entertainment pages. Sport is also an unmentionable topic.

Considering the political involvement of some of the participants in East End socialist activities, it would seem rather odd that these people should lose all political consciousness. However, the disregard of politics, as of any topic relating to mobility, hierarchy, progress and change, makes sense as an attempt to avoid any infringement of the time boundaries developed by participants.

The possibility of meaningful engagement in politics as an alternative life to the Centre is obviously extremely remote for people over seventy years old, poor, disabled and socially outcast. Nevertheless some external options are viable, and demand constant reference and response. There are two possible changes in the participants' way of life which might be opted for and which would mean an overall alteration of their state. The one, which is very uncommon, is the possibility of living with the children. The other, which is a daily temptation as well as a menace, is the possibility of being admitted into an old age home.

As the former option is open to very few participants, it will be discussed only briefly. Invariably there is an overriding rejection of the idea and in the light of the renunciation phenomenon this is hardly surprising. The following description taken from the participants' bulletin *News and Views* puts this reaction in a nutshell:

> One afternoon we were entertained by Mr B. with an unusual task. We were all asked to become Marjorie Proops. Letters had been sent to him asking for advice on various subjects and he read them out to the members and we had to give our opinion on them ... The best letter of all was certainly the one dealing with the question 'Could I go to live with my children?' I have been a member for many years and have heard shouting and talking galore, but the resounding 'NO' to that question was decisive and final and what a discussion followed.

As opposed to this possibility, old age homes are often a compulsory measure taken by family and/or social workers. This makes the imminence of admission an ominous indication of the final and critical curtailment of independence and autonomy. The forces involved in forestalling this threat and in making it cognitively invalid are varied, and to trace them an analysis of a few cases will be given. As the subject of old age homes impregnates the everyday life of the Centre, it is impossible to give a full and detailed account of its dominance and effects. However, some facets of this will be explored in the following discussion.

As old age homes are both a temptation, to alleviate increasing daily problems of coping, and a threat to one's freedom to choose and decide, they present a fundamental existential issue for potential residents. Invariably, the tendency in the Centre is towards a complete rejection of the idea of entering a home, but this is not a straightforward resolution, nor is it an easy attitude to take in the face of the stark facts of disablement, senility and general deterioration. The social processes through which this final view is moulded are complex and sometimes rather devious, for they inevitably involve factors beyond the participants' control.

One dominant factor is the approach to the subject taken by social workers and the impact of the way in which they present their view is crucial. As a whole, social workers in the Centre and in the Marlsden team adopted a strong and consistent line, discouraging old age home applications and, except in the cases of extremely confused, disorientated people, rejecting such institutions as an acceptable solution to the problems of old age. In effect, participants lean on this unequivocal attitude to assist them in sorting out the various considerations involved in reaching a decision.

A discussion on the subject held in the Jewish Blind Society centre produced initially mixed, indecisive reactions. Participants vacillated between the arguments for and against, and at one stage seemed to have embarked upon an altercation. The supervisor who led the group silenced the members and told them the story of a 'home application' case and its consequences. It concerned a woman who constantly and bitterly complained about the state of her accommodation. She was paid a home visit by the supervisor to inspect the situation, and having seen her squalid, mice-infested, dingy, high flat he decided that there was no other solution but to acknowledge the urgency of her application and to accept it. She was admitted to one of the Board's homes and at first seemed to be content enough, but gradually she changed her mind and requested a return to her home and independence. As the flat had already been sold by the council, her wish could not be granted and, being in a state of despair and frustration, she escaped from the home in an attempt to take possession of her flat. She was caught and sent back to the institution, where she showed accelerated deterioration towards senility and apathy.

A complete and lengthy silence followed, and an unmistakable change of attitude began to be expressed. Condemnation of the idea of old age homes was pronounced, and a flow of personal experiences was related by the members. They summoned up the harshness and severity of institutional life as opposed to the freedom and autonomy found in a home environment. As one of the participants said, 'I prefer to die in my own bed rather than have all the comfort in the world in an old age home.'

A few days later one of the most popular women participants was admitted into a home at her own request. She had been living on her own, and being severely disabled was confined to her room most of the time. A series of blackouts and falls clinched the realization that her unattended state was not only extremely inconvenient, but also rather perilous. A farewell presentation was made to her and she departed from the Centre in tears.

Rumours from her institution reached the Centre that she had become a constant source of trouble to the staff and to her fellow residents, and a few weeks later she was seen again happily rambling around the Centre. It was established that she left the home without any notification to the staff, and decided to return to the Centre. Her institutional phase was entirely overlooked by the participants, and the whole subject was not mentioned again. However, it was obvious evidence of the superiority of the Centre to an institution.

A debate which followed a film show on old age homes demonstrates the course and variety of reactions to the possibility of admission. The film itself presented a realistic, unmitigated picture of the life and the residents in a Jewish Welfare Board home. The disorientation, confusion, incontinence and lack of independence so common in old age homes were clearly featured, and the impression one got was of a place of gloom and doom, with no hope of improvement and no contact with the outside world.

The impact on the spectators was in sharp contrast to the usual afternoon jubilant, light-hearted atmosphere. The immediate response was that euthanasia should become a compulsory measure to obviate the possibility of people getting into such a state. This was followed by statements from a few participants who described their voluntary work for residents in homes and hospitals. A subsequent reaction was a self-reassuring assertion made by a number of participants that the age structure in old age homes is over ninety and homogeneous.

All this was obviously meant to show that the social and age distance between the Centre people and old age home residents is still wide enough to remove the immediate threat of identification with a typical institutionalized population. This firm cognitive obliteration was shattered by a woman participant who claimed to have met a schoolmate of hers in an old age home. The resident friend was in possession of all her faculties and she entered the institution after being refused attention by her family.

The first response was a complete upheaval in the anti-homes mood. Participants could not praise too highly the facilities and care provided by the staff in institutions and some of them even went further, declaring their intention to put their names on the waiting list for a vacancy.

This impulse was reversed when a number of participants suggested that a home application is not considered on the merits of the case, but according to the extent of influence and power the candidate can exert in order to forward his case. This insinuation was firmly denied by the supervisor, but it seemed that not many participants took heed of him. One of them concluded the discussion by saying, 'If two people in the same state were recommended to a home, one by me and the other by Sir Charles Clore, who would be accepted?'

The knowledge that none of the Centre attendants, by virtue of this very fact, was remotely related to an influential figure in the Jewish community, made the idea of family influence to get an elderly member into a home practically inconceivable. Thus the barrier was again erected, but this time on social rather than on personal foundations. The discussion ended with a reiterated disapproval of institutional life, and what was almost a solemn pledge not to let anybody submit to it.

The highly precarious nature of these boundaries was clearly demonstrated in the course of a direct confrontation with an old age home. This occurred when the Centre's concert group (participants who gave musical shows to other establishments for the elderly) performed at one of the Board's homes for infirm people.

At the beginning, facing the unresponsive, immobile residents, the members of the cast seemed to be embarrassed and lost. Gradually some of them started defining the situation by remarking that surely the average age of those residents was over ninety and that only at that age could one reach such a degree of degeneration.

To a remark from a member of the staff that one of the residents was only sixty-four, a member of the group retorted, 'I still prefer my poor flat to this luxury hotel with all these people around.' Other participants added that they would not wish even their enemies to live in such a place and that all the modern facilities available at the institution could not compensate for the Centre atmosphere and their independence. Questions addressed to the staff while being shown around the building were phrased in terms of 'us' and 'them', as if there was no basis for identification with the inmates.

Undoubtedly, the role of entertainers alleviated the poignancy of the encounter, for it allowed the participants to draw an acceptably clear line between them and the residents. Indeed, on the way back to the Centre the only subject of conversation was the professional aspect of the performance, and plans for future shows and appearances. The visit in fact stimulated further activities by the group.

The negation of old age homes as a viable alternative stems not only from the realization that life in a total institution necessarily involves a severe curtailment of independence, and thus inertia and withdrawal, but also from the knowledge that, as one of the participants put it, 'They are places to die in, not to live in.' Of course, death is the constant challenge. A complex of attitudes and practices were developed in the Centre to arrest time and to defy the idea of death. Some of these are the subject of what follows.

The ultimate reality

Participants are naturally well aware of impending death, considering their age and state of health, but this is rarely manifested in straightforward verbal and symbolic references. In order to appreciate their manner of coping with death, something must be said about the ways in which they perceive departure from the Centre.

In their analysis of total institutions for the incurable, Miller and Gwynne (1972, p.80) state:

To lack any actual or potential role that confers a positive social status in the wider society is tantamount to being socially dead. To be admitted to one of these institutions is to enter a kind of limbo in which one has been written off as a member of society but is not yet physically dead.

For the Centre people there was no need to become inmates in order to be virtually socially dead. The limbo state encapsulates most of the characteristics of this roleless position, and the Centre's boundaries, reinforced by the erasure of other realities, merely reinforce it. The social vacuum produced is filled by a new vision from which the idea of change into another, alternative world is eliminated. Any move away from the Centre is repressed. Therefore, leaving the Centre, and death, although different to the outsider, are elided. Both are disregarded by the participants, just as the Centre and its inhabitants are ignored by the outside. Impending death is not the final social disengagement, but rather another form of departing from the Centre into a changeable and insecure world.

The participants know this world as a place where they were socially buried, and also as an area in which physical death is omnipresent. A great number of them were at death's gate before entering the Centre and a few of them who were declared clinically dead at some stage enjoyed a narrow escape. Apart from heart attacks and other physical afflictions, a number of participants attempted to take their own lives, and so to some death appeared a possible release. Most of the participants were surrounded by other people passing away. The juxtaposition between death and the outside world can be seen in the following case:

Joel, a widower of a reputable well-known local politician, and suffering from a serious heart condition, regarded his stay in the Centre as a transitory phase until his financial affairs were sorted out, enabling him to transfer himself to a hotel for the elderly. In the meantime he isolated himself from other participants and behaved in a cantankerous manner to staff.

When eventually Joel left the Centre he was rarely mentioned by participants and even the very few close friends whom he seemed to make there managed to regroup without any noticeable disarray. A few days later Joel died from a heart attack in his hotel. The staff were more obviously upset than the participants, since for the latter he was non-existent as soon as he left the Centre. The few reactions drew attention to the association between his death and his departure, pointing out the seeming consequential link. A number of participants commented that by leaving the Centre Joel gave up his last lease on life. The Centre had provided a constant source of stimulation, even if he did not accept it. Some even suggested that his expressed resentment of the Centre did not reflect his real attitude, and that deep down he recognized it as his only significant world. His departure did not seem to be relevant to his judgment.

The connection between death and departure was also demonstrated on the death of a male participant, whose wife was a participant-volunteer. The only subject widely discussed amongst participants was whether or not the widow would continue her participation, as there was a possibility that she would have to go to work to support herself. The dead husband represented a definite departure and as such was beyond mentioning, whereas the wife, being in a precarious situation, aroused uncertainties and speculation.

Another incident occurred when, after being refused a diet meal with his wife, a participant walked out and committed suicide by electrocuting himself on the nearby railway line. I heard no mention of this tragedy from any of the participants, and the case only came to my knowledge accidentally, when browsing through the participants' files.

A member of staff who died in a fire was not referred to as a dead person. One might have imagined that the girl was still alive and working somewhere else. In conversations and daily encounters the death of participants was rarely mentioned. The Centre magazine, *News and Views*, would have ignored deaths of participants had it not been for the obituaries written by members of staff.

Nevertheless, sometimes an unavoidable confrontation occurs, producing reactions ranging from denial to full acceptance. Denial is the most common, acceptance occurring when people are obliged to contemplate the realistic possibility of their own death. Denial takes the form of, 'it won't happen to me', and in many respects it resembles the invalidation mechanism already discussed. Indeed, the menacing contingency of a transfer to an old age home is closely associated with death. Participants who visited such institutions often remarked on the readiness for death expressed by the inmates. The state of these inmates was sharply contrasted to that ruling in the Centre.

As death is the main reason for leaving the Centre, the association between the two is reinforced. Participants who were pushed, mainly in discussion groups taken by the staff, to contemplate the pros and cons of going into an institution were adamant that they would prefer death. Furthermore, some demanded euthanasia, or threatened suicide.

Yet confrontation with death was inevitable. Death in the outside world was talked about as if it happened to a separate category of people. Thus a participant who described the extreme social isolation prevailing in 'tower blocks' and related two cases of people who were found dead in the unvisited flats after having been ignored by their neighbours, referred to them as 'them old folk' or 'that old man'. Another participant stated that once he became old he would commit suicide. He was well over seventy and suffered from terminal cancer.

This denial sometimes reaches the point where people unwittingly overlook their own terminal disease. A man suffering from multiple sclerosis told a discussion group on euthanasia that it should be applied to people with no hope, 'but, thank God, I am lucky as my illness is not terminal'. A few days later he called me aside and apologized for the 'stupid mistake I made by saying that my illness is not terminal, I realize now that it is'.

The course of the discussion on euthanasia is significant for the understanding of the subject of death in the Centre. It was held in conjunction with the members of the Jewish Blind Society day centre, who unanimously took the view that euthanasia was a positively justified measure in the case of incurable diseases.[5] The Centre participants, however, having been reluctant to start the discussion at all, varied in their opinion and there seemed to be a definite discomfort and restlessness amongst them.

One participant argued that 'nobody really wants to die'. A proponent of euthanasia, who was asked to substantiate his argument, started a vivid description of his frequent visits to a home for the incurable, where he had witnessed deformed and severely handicapped people desperately trying to establish some contact with their surroundings. He was describing a young man, a victim of a car accident, whose brain was hardly functioning and whose movements were uncontrollable, when a few participants started heckling and eventually shouted him down. Alan, a leading figure, angrily rebuked him for discussing 'things which we are not interested in and anyway are irrelevant to the discussion'. Others joined in demanding that such 'horrible stories' should not be allowed in the Centre, where people are meant to forget and relax.

Alan who had kept quiet until the incident, now took over and with the full attention of the rest told the story of his father's death. Suffering from a long illness which left him bedridden and inflicted constant pain and confusion, the father in his periods of awareness and clarity reiterated emphatically that he did not wish to die and that no man-devised method of terminating life should be administered to him.

The impact of this story became immediately noticeable and more and more participants seconded Alan's view that euthanasia is an act against the most fundamental trait of human nature – the will to live. Seemingly this reaction arose from the genuine effect of the story and the desire to support Alan. Nevertheless, another dramatic incident made up the minds of the last of the doubters.

One of the participants, suffering from cancer of the throat, a man admired by all for his struggle to belittle his own plight and to cheer up other people, walked out when a Jewish Blind Society member put the case for euthanasia for terminal illnesses. The reaction amongst the Centre's participants was unequivocal. Angry demands to stop the discussion, which should not have been held in the first place, were voiced. Bringing up the subject had upset and distressed participants 'who are trying to forget all about it'. And, indeed, that was the end of the session.

Group pressure operated in other instances of direct confrontation with death. The faith-healer (see 'Alternative realities') who started his talk by relating his spiritual experience as a result of his wife's death was also heckled and jeered at by Alan and his friends, an act which gained the full backing of the other participants even from those who usually were known to be at odds with Alan. The speaker was bluntly accused of making participants unhappy by reminding them of the very subject they were trying to forget. As Alan and Joel remarked, 'We think about it enough when we come home and see the four walls around us.'

The borderline between the Centre and the world in which death prevails is maintained by participants with respect also to personal sorrow and the aftermath of bereavement. Social workers often remarked on the 'miraculous effect' of the Centre on the recently bereaved. Sometimes a few weeks' interval between a spouse's

death and admission to the Centre are sufficient for the newcomer
to get over his grief and participate fully in the Centre's life.

Outsiders frequently commented on the apparent indifference
shown by participants to the death of a close relation or friend. In
fact, participants are trying not to contaminate the Centre with
their personal anguish. Thus a woman whose best friend died
refrained from attending the Centre for a few days because 'I could
only make them unhappy.' Conversely, a participant whose
brother-in-law died 'took an hour off for the funeral', but otherwise abstained from mentioning the 'mishap', and did not let it
interfere with his usual Centre activities which included singing and
dancing.

Participants who do mention death are invariably regarded as
acting improperly and strangely. A woman who approached one of
the participants in his capacity as a committee member and asked
him who would bury her when her time came, sent her on to a
member of staff, speeded by a look of disgust and remarks on her
unbalanced behaviour.

However, one social enclave in the Centre was reserved for
direct encounters with the occurrence of death. This was the
'therapy group'. The conception of the Centre as a therapeutic
environment was a significant element in the social workers' view,
and a special group was set up to help participants in coping with
recent bereavements or severe loneliness. People were invited indi-
vidually by the supervisor to take part in the discussions. Members
were people who complained of unhappiness and depression,
together with others interested in 'helping' them.

Although conducted by the supervisor, the procedure was
informal. The only significant rule was that of confidentiality. No
information should be allowed to leak from the group to non-
members. This contrasted with the normal lack of internal barriers
in the Centre, and consequently provoked interest and rumours.
The fact that participants were encouraged to express their individuality instead of submerging their differences and identities was
also a novelty, and, unsurprisingly, the possibility of breaking out
of the Centre's mould was both intriguing and threatening.

One of the first subjects discussed was bereavement, and the
response was at first no more than an extension of the regular attitude in the Centre. Members refused to talk freely, and when asked
to express their feelings used clichés designed to evade the issue.

They disagreed strongly with the supervisor's suggestion that at one stage of the bereavement process a reaction of anger towards the deceased sets in. The impression they gave was rather of complete disengagement from the dead, accompanied by no more than formal expressions of sorrow and distress.

The only other taboo subject was homosexuality (and one is at liberty to speculate on the intrinsic association between the two topics). People went into the most intimate details of their sex life, the delicate fabric of the love-hate relationship with their spouses, and even discussed the poignant detachment from their children, but remained closed on these two issues.

On the rare unplanned occasion when the occurrence of death did penetrate the therapy group, there was a noticeable difference between the attitude of the members and the normal attitude of detachment. When one of the members died, someone suggested that they observe a minute's standing silence in his memory. This was accepted unquestioningly, but no eulogies were volunteered. Instead, members used the fact that the deceased had experienced bad relationships with his son as a starting point for a discussion on children's attitudes towards the elderly.

At the time of the silence the usual afternoon sounds of jubilation seeped through from the nearby dining hall into the rest room which accommodated the therapy group meeting. The contrast seemed to be so sharp that the supervisor asked the members to wait a little whilst he rushed to halt the merriment for a minute. When he returned the period of silence was already over and the members proceeded with the discussion.

On another occasion, when Joel died and one of the members asked the group to stand for a minute in silence, the suggestion was questioned on the grounds that Joel was not a group member. The matter was finally resolved by standing in commemoration of Joel's pro-Israeli activities, for which he was renowned in the Centre. Thus the event of his death was divorced from association with the Centre reality, and linked to the outside world.

This silent commemoration was not practised in other areas of the Centre life, and it is quite significant that the members of the group established, however reluctantly and cautiously, a corner where the taboo subject of death could be touched. This was undoubtedly connected to the unique nature of the group in the Centre, as a recognized place to probe the outside life of participants.

Nevertheless, feelings of loss and grief cannot be entirely regulated, and as much as participants accept the general rule that death
should be eliminated from the Centre world, there are occasions
when personal anguish demands expression. Even then people are
careful to keep the unwritten rules. A woman whose friend – also a
participant – had died the day before wanted to talk about him to
an interested acquaintance in the Centre. She took her aside and
out of earshot, in an unfrequented part of the upper hall, they
started conversing in low voices about the deceased. This was a
calculated effort to disengage the conversation from the general
setting of the Centre. The two women had been taking part in the
usual morning gathering of Alan's group, which in many ways
represented the epitome of the Centre's values (see 'Differentiations'). After their talk the women rejoined the group and no
further reference to the interruption was made.

Even a newcomer to the Centre managed to sense the borderline
between the Centre reality and personal engrossment with grief.
She was admitted to the Centre after the death of her son in a road
accident, and carried with her a book in which was one of the
poems,[6] referring to a possible restoration of the relationship
between the living and the dead, that gave her much comfort and
consolation. This book was not shown to any of the participants
and only members of staff were made aware of its meaning to her.

Participants who claimed to have had spiritualist experiences
usually gingerly confined their references to the matter to discussions and meetings directly germane to the subject. Thus a man was
convinced that he had been guided by his late wife in his daily life.
Furthermore, he maintained that several pleasing events had been
engineered by the intervention of his wife in the other world. His
evidence, which was put to a discussion group on religion, was
dismissed as unsubstantiated coincidences. Another participant,
who insisted that she had witnessed an apparition of her deceased
husband, was persuaded by members of another discussion group
on the supernatural that it was an hallucination caused by the
emotional stress of her husband's death.

The fact that no death actually occurred at the Centre helped to
buttress its cognitive elimination from the Centre reality. At the
same time the realization that participants are not safeguarded in
the world outside was significant in the building up of the pressure
to extend the Centre's activities and to provide more warden-

controlled accommodation for participants. The implicit belief that the Centre is a death-proof environment should not be dismissed as an obvious logical fallacy. The social mechanisms developed to construct the inadmissibility of death into the Centre had their own coherent plausibility and together with the erasure of the past and the invalidation of other realities, made the ultimate reality irrelevant to the existence of the Centre.

The cognitive denial of death completes the reconstruction of the Centre as an alternative reality to the outside and of the way some basic premises relating to time are eliminated from its conceived order of events. Thus the Centre has become a focus for the development of a counterpoise to the social seclusion and rejection which were experienced by its participants and which pushed them into attendance. The limbo state imposed by society was transformed into a sanctuary, where inhabitants have chosen to forget and obliterate their previous social world whilst constructing an alternative reality possessing many characteristics which reverse those of the outside world.

The revision of the past contains two complementary elements: the creation of a continuous, selected, collective past experience, closely related to the Centre, and the elimination of all other dividing, unequal and irrelevant factors. This common ground is defended by invalidating other realities which might supersede the Centre.

All these are merely prerequisites and to a certain extent by-products of a new content of time. The constitution of the time perspective as constructed by participants broaches a whole gamut of questions relating to the nature of the connection between events, the conduct of behaviour, and the social structure dominating it.

4 Constituting the Centre time

The arrest of progress, the repetitive nature of events and the selective erasure of the past are also predominant characteristics of the interaction between members. Yet there is one essential difference between their operation in marking the relations between the Centre and the outside world and their place in moulding the relationships with the Centre. We have seen them in their negative guise of invalidation, negation, elimination, etc., aiming at establishing what the Centre is not. The time universe in the Centre itself, embedded in behaviour and attitudes, has, on the other hand, a more positive function, indicating rather what the Centre world is.

Participants have created in the Centre a mirror image of the outside world. This is a system of principles and a code of behaviour built upon the realization that as care and concern are not to be found outside, the Centre community should create its own substitutes. The main features of this system of care, and its implications for the conception of time in the Centre, will be the subject of the following two sections. This will be followed by a discussion of the relations between this system and the other daily activities of the Centre – again with reference to the time universe of the participants.

The idea of care

The distant past, mainly East End childhood, is often evoked in a manner suggesting that mutual aid and community care predominated in early relationships, whereas disregard and desertion were the prominent features of later life. Furthermore, the onus of obtaining help and concern in the East End was not on the recipient, but was volunteered because of people's basic moral attitudes. In contrast, help in later years was merely a function of self-interest or connections. Care was not rendered any longer on the basis of need, but rather because of influence and pressure.

Thus participants attributed the rarity of their visits to Israel – the only acceptable alternative reality to the Centre – not to shortage of money, but to the absence of people willing to look after them during the journey and to help them out in difficult situations caused by their physical disabilities. In such ways, participants constitute a picture of an unhelpful, uncaring environment which makes the outside world extremely insecure and threatening for people who cannot fend for themselves.

Doctors and members of the helping professions who are expected and supposed to help, pay no attention to their elderly patients and clients. Moreover, even friends, who used to come to the rescue when needed, are unable or unwilling to show concern. Participants lament that as this foundation for friendship has been lost, friendships are discontinued. Suggestions by members of staff that friendship could be maintained on the basis of shared past experiences, and coloured by reminiscences, were dismissed as 'unrealistic', for a 'shared past' as such has no bearing.

The realization that there is nobody in the outside world who would bother to offer genuine help, was accentuated by the derogatory interpretations given to certain forms of social concern enjoyed by elderly people in everyday life (see 'The end of involvement'). Gestures such as offering a seat on a bus, carrying a shopping bag or help in crossing the road, were often viewed as social supports for the inferior position to which elderly people are subjected and, therefore, as humiliating acts of charity. The reaction of one participant was, 'This is for me the last proof that I am not a human being any more.'

Family relationships, especially those between spouses, are also revised in terms of the element of care embedded in their conduct. Former wives were judged in terms of the devotion they had shown their husbands. Widows in particular tended to attach great importance to the use of a selected terminology of care whilst describing their former family life. Some confessed that there had been no love between them and their late husbands, but instead their relationship had been one of infinite care and boundless concern. As one woman said, 'I have never loved my husband, but I got to really care for him. I wouldn't touch a hair on his head.' This was not an apologetic attitude by any means and women did not feel shame or reserve in admitting lack of love. On the other hand, a number of them seemed rather proud to stress that, although circumstances forced them to look after their sick and disabled spouses, the element of care in the relationship was entirely voluntary, a result of moral conviction rather than social commitment.

Outside the family, situations of seeming equality were frequently mentioned as arenas for rendering help (see 'Revising the past'). Service in the army and hospitalization are the most notable examples and participants are only too glad to elaborate on their care experiences in those settings, regardless of the obvious coercive element in the situation. Accounts of saving a fellow soldier or another patient were widespread in the Centre, and were often associated with the general framework of apparent egalitarianism surrounding the case. A typical example of such juxtaposition, interlinking equality and care, is the following story told by a woman participant who had just returned to the Centre from a long stay in hospital.

In the same breath she described two elements of hospital life. The first concerned a game played by patients. All were given a trade, occupation or profession and they had to convey this information to the other participants in the game by charade. The second incident occurred when she had prevented a patient in her ward from committing suicide, and consequently won the appreciation and the thanks of the staff. The connection between the reversed role situation, indicating a complete freedom from social constraints, and the personal act of help, was obviously in the woman's mind.

Care became the declared foundation for establishing relationships with other people. The ultimate expression of this is reached when care and concern result in marriage. Participants maintained that as care is a vital, indispensable element in their lives, they would be inclined to base their new marital life upon it. Thus a participant stated his wish to marry his girl friend 'after she has proven her feelings towards me by looking after me when I am in hospital'. Another participant explained his desire to remarry by the need to be taken care of in his later years. Again, there is an explicit contrast to the commonly accepted idea in the outside world that love is a necessary, if not essential, prerequisite for marriage.

Concentrating on the value of care has altered their outlook on life in general. This was evident when participants responded to the hypothetical problem of 'reliving one's life'. Without exception they emphasized that if they were to lead their lives again they would render more help to people and devote all their material and spiritual resources to pursuing this mission. A leading participant summed up this view by asserting, 'If I had any regrets in my life it is the fact that I couldn't help other people more than I did.'

This self-criticism should not be interpreted as implying that participants had not tried to help. On the contrary, they could not stress too strongly that only circumstances had forced them to withhold help, and instances of self-sacrifice and going out of one's way to help provided a common topic of conversation in the Centre. This underlines the conviction that their stay in the Centre is merely a restitution rendered by society for previous 'good behaviour' and that therefore feelings of receiving charity or mercy are unwarranted. Thus, the shame attached to attending the Centre is removed by seeing attendance in terms of the imbalance in over-all reciprocal relationships between them and society. Suggestions that joining the Centre resulted from boredom, loneliness and financial and physical difficulties seemed to be irrelevant in the light of the real main objective of attendance – rendering help. What might be seen as an ideology of reciprocity between the participants and the outside world is merely an indication of the intricate relationship with other realities. Although the dominant characteristic of such a relationship is disengagement and negation, the participants did not rid themselves completely of the various links and associations with the external world.

This ideology enables people to see themselves, from the inception of their participation, not as mere passive recipients, but mainly as contributors and helpers. Some of them in their conclusive interview with the social worker, before actual attendance, expressed their wish to be useful and insisted on being regarded first and foremost as helpers rather than participants.

Thus, people who were to all intents and purposes potential participants preferred to enter the Centre in the capacity of volunteers or to offer certain services as an excuse for participation. Many strongly denied that their attendance was necessitated by insuperable difficulties in pre-Centre conditions. They had come to help other people and to look after the needy. Other participants used to add that as they had been helped recently, and managed to overcome their own hardships, they thought it only fair to come to the Centre in order to use their experience to assist others.

This care consciousness was made a central factor in applying to the Centre. Members of staff emphasized the readiness and the ability of a candidate to make himself useful in the course of his future participation. Social workers' reports seemed to place high importance on the assessment of a client as a potential helper and those who showed conspicuous willingness enjoyed a high degree of esteem. In this respect the concept of care has become a major criterion for participation and as such a major theme in the relationship between staff and members, creating a comprehensive framework for communication as well as a source of tension and conflict (see 'Patterns of help').

The members of the committee of participants were appointed by the supervisor on the grounds of their seeming willingness and ability to be of help in the Centre. Participants rarely questioned this system of representation and tended to accept the supremacy of the principle of help over any form of franchise. An attempt to apply this principle as a possible basis for tightening relationships between the Centre and the participants' families was made occasionally, but the call to relatives, especially children, to come and help produced no response. In many instances it was not passed on by the participants to the people concerned, in other cases the call was neglected or met by blunt refusal. Such rebuffs provided added corroboration of the careless attitude of society, and a heightened contrast to the reality in the Centre.

The criteria of care penetrated every aspect of relationships in the Centre. Participants judged members of staff on the merits of their actual help, and tended to belittle vague gestures of sympathy offered instead of offers of tangible, purposeful help. Thus participants rarely refer to members of staff in terms of their official capacity, but rather in relation to their appreciation of the help rendered. Members of staff who for one reason or another do not live up to the expectations of participants are either deliberately ignored by them – e.g. 'forgetting' his name – or referred to disparagingly. Such attitudes are facilitated by the loose definition of staff hierarchy and roles (see 'The running of the Centre').

Similarly, though in inverse fashion, members of staff adopted this criterion as a main form of reference to participants. The new supervisor absorbed this predominating value within a few days of his arrival, and built his own evaluation scale in terms of help. Thus in staff meetings and encounters with participants one would hear him speaking of a participant 'who is willing to help', or another 'who is just talking but is not doing very much to help'. He applied similar criteria to members of staff. In the supervisor's opinion his underlings should be regarded and treated as patients, and indeed much of their interchange revolved around the effect of their personal emotional problems on their work, and it was not uncommon at staff meetings to hear self-exposure and confession, analysed by all present. This view of others as objects for help was also the prevailing attitude towards outsiders, especially volunteers who came to the Centre to help. Their activities were regarded as a form of therapy for themselves, and hence instead of being regarded exclusively as helpers, they were often treated as 'cases' seeking help.

Staff members also became subject to the care system, by being recipients of help from participants. Thus a former social worker in the Centre was described to me as a 'wounded Israeli soldier who was helped by us to learn English'. The fact that he was in a position of authority in the Centre for quite a while was overlooked. A series of discussions led by a new member of staff on the taboo subject of religion was attended in order to help him in his first steps in the new job (see 'Alternative realities').

The main arena for participants' direct help to staff was the therapy group (see 'The ultimate reality'). All the members of the group explained their participation was meant to help the leader of the group – the supervisor – to gain a better understanding of old people and their problems and thereby to assist him in carrying out what seemed to them to be his vocational interest in helping the elderly. Some of them added that as the Centre is the most important thing in their lives, they would not hesitate to contribute to its success and smooth running by advising members of staff.

A member of the therapy group who expressed her distress at hearing incessantly 'things I am trying to forget in the Centre – things like being old and sick and unwanted' was dissuaded by other members of the group from quitting as 'we know it is very unpleasant for all of us, but we have got to do everything to help this devoted young man – without people like him we would be in greater trouble.' The supervisor himself encouraged this outlook by explicitly asking for help in assessing the activities in the Centre, and the staff, and in planning specific matters such as a talk on the

Centre in the Jewish Welfare Board's head office.

Direct help to staff was also given on a regular basis in the handling of discussion groups, serving of lunches, compiling of the daily register of attendance, etc. Special events which seemed to necessitate participants' help did not pass unheeded either. The merger with the Jewish Blind Society's day centre, despite the strong opposition expressed by participants to its implementation, did not encounter complete lack of co-operation as 'we the participants must realize that the staff is trying to cope with grave financial difficulties and this Jewish Blind Society business is their only hope to overcome them and we have got to do everything to help.'

The conception of help and care as an overriding value in the Centre was expressed on innumerable occasions, and I cannot over-emphasize the verbal attention given to it. In the opening of a general meeting of participants, one of the committee members delivered a speech on the virtues of help and on the need to render it unconditionally. The speech, which at times reached a high emotional pitch, described the speaker's desire to centre his life around helping his fellow participants and urged them to follow his example. This was greeted by cheers and applause.

There were very few participants who did not mention the will to help as their chief motive in joining the Centre. Help was not a means of alleviating other people's hardships, but an end in itself, regardless of the recipients. A participant who came to the Centre because 'it has always been my desire in life to help' confessed that he had had no interest whatsoever in the participants as objects for personal interaction. In fact, quite the opposite – he often used derogatory terms ranging from 'insignificant' and 'primitive' to 'animals', to describe them. Nevertheless, both parties chose to ignore the terminology in favour of a more relevant viewpoint, namely that as he was willing to help and was in need of help himself, he deserved to be an integral part of the community.

A sense of belonging to the Centre could be gained only by immersion in the care system. A participant who tried to explain this said, 'I want to be one of the boys, I want to be a helper of a helper of a helper.' Another participant, about to set off for home, said to the supervisor, 'I really feel this place is myself. I have been working like a dog all day, helping everybody.'

Care is also often seen as the ultimate justification for enjoying the Centre facilities. A woman who said a wish to help was the prime reason for her participation, decided to leave the Centre after realizing that due to ill health, she could no longer maintain the necessary level of activity. As she put it, 'I can't be of any service to the Centre any more.' Another participant, severely disabled and consequently incapable of most forms of help requiring physical exertion, claimed jokingly that 'I am here to instruct other people how to help.' Thus the total commitment to the idea of care may cause problems when one is no longer in a position to practise what is preached.

Participants who were 'caught' doing nothing were often treated critically. The usual reaction was apologetic, people perhaps blaming temporary incapacity to help on emotional distress, or physical relapse. In some cases the critic was accused of misinterpreting the situation. 'I was listening to his troubles'; or, 'I was trying to think how to help and what to do.'

Even ordinary daily greetings revolve around the motif of care and questions such as 'Are you all right today?' or 'Have you been looked after well hy him?' (addressed to a wife in a wheelchair pushed by her husband) substitute for the normal 'How are you?' A detailed answer is expected which in most cases develops into a conversation concerning the problems of the people involved.

Help as a coherent ideology was expressed by a few participants, of whom the most notable was Joseph. In his background Joseph deviates considerably from the picture of the typical participant. He is Indian born, an ex-business man, university educated and the possessor of extensive general knowledge on Judaism, other religions and the sciences. Being separated from his wife he had chosen to lead a life free of commitments and ties, to claim no social security benefits and to refuse fixed accommodation, spending his nights in Salvation Army hostels, tube stations, parks and church crypts. Joseph explained these self-imposed hardships as 'an experiment in survival'. Being certain that the scourges of modern technology and progress will end up in a worldwide calamity leaving people homeless and starving, he decided to show the world ways of surviving with a minimum of food and sleep. This mission was to be written up as a book, its theme being the need to care for other people. The origins of this ideology are immaterial to the fact that Joseph found the Centre reality the only one suitable for propagating and practising his ideas which, to a certain extent, might have developed within its care context. The conversion of the stigma into stigmata of martyrdom – the creation of a 'heaven' populated by 'saints' as opposed to the 'hellish outside world – was perhaps most epitomized by Joseph who coupled qualities of extreme asceticism and a fervent denial of the world.

Joseph's catastrophe theory suggests another characteristic of the concept of care – the universality of the need for help. Everybody is liable to be affected and should be entitled to help merely on the merits of his needs. Difference in class, creed or race is irrelevant (for a more detailed discussion on the idea of equality in the Centre see 'Revising the past'). Thus whilst discussing coloured people in the area, participants carefully distinguished their hostility to muggers and molesters, and the care relationship they enjoyed with some of their neighbours. A woman whose house was ransacked by a coloured youth, described how she was the only neighbour to help an elderly woman from Jamaica who came to visit her family, and owing to language difficulties could not communicate with anybody.

Another participant expressed his admiration for a social worker who came from a well-known affluent family, but who visited his house and was prepared, as he put it, 'to scrape the floor for me'. In his view 'this was a real example of genuine help, not because she is a social worker, but because she is a human being.'

No difficulty should inhibit the rendering of help. An extreme example is a case which was described by a social worker as 'hopeless', and given the following assessment in a report:

'Visited Mr Y. in hospital in order to assess suitability for a mentally infirm home. Mr Y. was sitting in a chair in a dressing gown and looked very confused and had deteriorated very much since I last saw him at the Day Centre. He was not able to answer any of my questions coherently.'

Jonathan who had attended that interview with the social worker passed an entirely different opinion: 'He is clean and responsible and wouldn't prove any trouble in the Centre.'

Care is not only the ultimate aim of a participant, but is also a sole criterion for his appreciation – a criterion exceeding any other human quality. An argumentative, cantankerous participant who was much disliked by other participants was strongly defended by a member of the committee who said, 'I don't care what you lot say, but for me he is first and foremost a very good helper, never refuses to give a hand and this is the most important thing I can see in a person.' To the allegation that sometimes this defiant, insulting behaviour was intolerable, he answered that perhaps he was ill and that in that event it was their business to look after him. (For further references to the use of illness as a rationale for mis-behaviour see 'Guarding the system').

The desire to help should surpass any other feelings. This became evident when whilst listening to the entertainers singing 'A Yiddisha Mama' (see 'Revising the past') a few participants started crying. Immediately fellow members began to comfort them. A few of those 'helpers' remarked later that they wanted to cry as much as the rest, but the need to look after those who were already crying was stronger.

Life-long friendship is also put to the test of the care system. A and B, who had known each other from childhood and seemed to have established a fairly close relationship, were involved in a row over another participant, C, who was cared for by A. The conflict started when B bluntly accused C of being lazy, and although able to work, of seeking help under false pretences. This was denied by A and C. A demanded an apology from B, who refused to retract, and from then on not a word was exchanged between them. This dispute, apparently over labelling, really involved a difference in interpretation of the boundaries of the system, and their rigidity.

Participants who could no longer help developed severe guilty consciences. A member of the committee confessed that she could no longer live up to her own expectations, and asked the other members to accept her resignation. This was refused, and she was advised that the only way to alleviate these guilt feelings was to try and help more. The only alternative was to quit altogether. Even members of staff who occasionally fobbed off participants because of pressure of work, often experienced guilt and remorse.

This leads us to another item in the code of care – the right to help. The right to receive help is unconditional and so is the right to render it. People do not do 'favours' by helping nor should they expect a reward. It is their privilege to be a helper, and there is a widespread recognition in the Centre that relationships should be constructed in a way which would allow almost everybody, regard-less of physical and mental limitations, to enjoy this status. A situation may be fabricated to enable a participant to see himself in the position of a helper. A participant who suffered from the crippling after-effects of a stroke, was deliberately allowed by an able-bodied man to 'aid' and escort him downstairs, by holding his arm. The reversal of roles was obvious and yet evoked no amazement nor questioning, and participants who witnessed the incident just smiled at the differences in height between the two which made the man being 'helped' look like a child being led by an adult.

In a discussion of the desirable type of institutional care for the elderly, a suggestion was made that old age homes should cater for a mixed population of able-bodied and infirm residents. This would enable people to help each other and to bridge the differences between them. The idea, which won the applause of the audience, was described by a participant as a 'copy of our own Centre', and another one added, 'If there are no differences, people can't offer help, and this would be a great shame.'

Helping other people is the major ingredient in human happiness. A participant who made this point in a public talk added that happiness is merely the spiritual reward for having helped somebody.

The view that help is a prerequisite for meaningful human relationships was disseminated and reinforced through a number of channels. An articulate expression is to be found in verses written by Joseph to mark a visit to the Centre by a group of young volunteers:

> Modern youth is often maligned
> though jewels among them I often find.
> This week I met a willing band
> who gladly gave a helping hand.
> To give a breath of seasons cheer
> to folk whose own is not so near.
> To wish them well I've written this
> May they find a life of bliss.
> Free from worry and from pain
> Who knows when we meet again
> It's been pleasant meeting you
> Alas too soon we say 'adieu'.

A more general conception of care as one of the foundations of Joseph's idea of the 'golden age' to come is expressed in the following, written as a thanksgiving to the volunteers in a Salvation Army hostel:

Farewell folk that ease the plight
of lonely wanderers in the night
in trust of all were tables laid.
No thought of greed had staged a raid
Giving all the friendly hand
passing hopes of promised land.
The time comes soon when perverse seed
caters for all in pressing need
when all mankind the burdens share
and natures beauty is everywhere.
Then, the halt, the lame and meek
Not from strangers.succour to seek
Ancient wrongs are put to right
Hate, envy, greed no more a blight
Till that day dawns to ease your load
In goodwill could you spread the word
The love of many will cast out fears
Be sure that golden age is near.

This millennial vision, based on a division of the world into 'helpers' and 'non-helpers', is accentuated where religious people are concerned. The invalidation of religion as an alternative reality is largely due to the denial of expected help and concern by religious institutions and individuals, although one participant said, 'I wouldn't mind if non-religious people don't help, after all they don't have to practise what they never preached.' The general view is that as God does not help then there is no reason to believe in His existence. The value of care is seen as the basis for any genuine religion. Participants often expressed the view that the pivotal precept of all faith should be the principle of rendering care unconditionally. This theme was usually presented in terms of personal commitment. Statements such as, 'my religion is to help people', or, 'I pray in what I do for other people', were not uncommon.

The conviction that the principle of care should guide people's behaviour irrespective of their differences underlay judgments of external affairs. General subjects such as 'How to make the world a better place to live in' or 'Are the trips to the moon justified?' come back to this line of argument. The answer is to be sought in the intensification of care, and an increase in resources directed to help. Examples of individuals and institutions who do show concern were invariably acclaimed and taken as evidence that the idea of care could be materialized and implemented.

Examining the overall care ideology in the Centre, one can hardly avoid an analogy with a typical religious sectarian reaction to the world, consisting of denial and rejection of the world and the erection of rigid boundaries between members and non-members. This analogy will be elaborated upon later (see 'Initiation', 'Guarding the system').

Patterns of help

The way in which the idea of care is translated into patterns of behaviour in the Centre is governed by a number of norms. These relate to the nature and content of the actual help rendered, to the circumstances under which care is justified or unwarranted, and to the expected relationships between the manipulation of care and other aspects of the Centre world, especially those concerning the internal structure of power amongst participants.

The denial of self-pity and charitable attitudes (see 'Choice') makes the introduction of these elements into the care system unwelcome. Participants insisted emphatically that 'doing favours for the sake of it' and 'just sympathy' were not compatible with their ideal. With this exception, views on the subject of what care is were generally vague. People preferred describing an acceptable situation of care to specifying its ingredients. 'Paying attention' and 'looking after' were the commonest descriptions of the care situation. Metaphorical expressions, such as, 'I am like a father to him', or, 'we are all social workers here', were also often used.

Nevertheless, certain forms of help were more common and conspicuous than others, and as such became prototypes. To mention just a few: calling each other for lunch, making and serving tea, attempting to arrange transport for participants in urgent need, aiding the disabled in moving about the place, exchanging useful information on pensions and other benefits and entitlements, including tips on how to obtain these. Calls for help were rarely necessary, as it was a common procedure for participants to enquire as to the well-being of their fellow members, and a precise answer was expected. Moreover, a personal balance of reciprocity was not expected. Thus participants who were about to leave the

Centre for some reason still took an active interest in giving help, and so did participants who otherwise had very little contact with the people who enjoyed their attentions.

The most striking example of the non-mutuality of help is to be found in the offers made by participants to help other establishments such as old age homes, day centres and pensioners' clubs. The lack of positive response on the part of these organizations inhibited these initiatives, however, and with the exception of the concert party entertainment tour (discussed later), no care attempts extended beyond the territory of the Centre.

The expectation of direct reciprocity would, in any case, be senseless, given the extremely uneven distribution of the ability to help amongst the participants. A person's capability also varies at différent times. Certain participants became renowned for some specific types of help, and consequently established a position distinct from that of other, non-specialized participants. A former underwriter, who happened to be in fairly good health, could advise participants on legal matters, and also help shifting furniture, and assist the disabled. Other participants showed various degrees of versatility, all allocating their care according to needs. Thus, the 'specialists' did not exchange help among themselves, nor did they make their help conditional on a due reward. Instead their special abilities were used whenever necessary, according to the requirements of specific situations.

Perhaps the most significant characteristics of this attitude towards help is the lack of the element of personal achievement. Two examples may clarify the point. There were some considerable variations in the skill and competence of participants who were engaged in craft work. Nevertheless, not only did those who produced better articles instruct the less gifted participants and on occasions make the items for the completely incapacitated, but they also did not express much enthusiasm at the possibility of exhibiting their work in a special glass cabinet which was designed and built for that purpose. Such an act would have clearly demonstrated to outsiders the marked differences between participants and hence would have created a hierarchy of personal achievements. The other example is the playing of chess, when in a manner contradictory to the normal competitive spirit of the game, those about to win deliberately spoiled their own chances and enabled their opponent to draw, pretending that they were taking part in a teaching exercise. A public-speaking contest organized by members of staff was converted into a non-competitive therapeutic experiment. Contestants placed little value on the rhetorical qualities of the speeches, but rather on the significance of the fact that a participant with grave physical or mental handicaps managed to make them. Thus, in a semi-final between an eloquent contestant and a less articulate one, who had just left hospital after a series of heart attacks, the former was acknowledged to be the better speaker, but the latter won the applause of the audience, who commented on the remarkable recovery and high spirits indicated by the speech. Considering the high importance attached by participants in their pre-Centre situation to 'good education', represented by eloquence in the English language (see 'Disintegration'), the abandonment of such criteria was another facet of denying the worldly standards of esteem and respect in favour of the care system yardsticks. (For further discussion on the lack of the element of achievement in the Centre, see the following section.)

This denial of competitiveness is congruent with the notion that everyone gives and receives help, is a benefactor and beneficiary, a giver and recipient, at the same time, though not necessarily in respect of the same person. One cannot be a viable part of the system without accepting this duality, and one should be prepared for a swift switch of roles. This interplay does not allow for a distinctive dichotomy between 'helpers' and 'helped'.

The rules are waived in some cases, two categories of which are particularly instructive. The first exception is the relationship with outsiders, who usually do not submerge themselves in the Centre's life and, therefore, are not regarded as subject to the expected conduct of behaviour within the care system. Thus a participant whose tape recorder was repaired by a visitor immediately said, 'You looked after me, now I will look after you', and rushed to serve him tea. This insistence on direct reciprocity seldom emerged in the relationships between participants. It would have been incongruous with the general lack of mutuality, and incompatible with the awareness that help is not rendered as a part of exchange between individuals, but rather on the basis of compliance with an overall code of norms.

The other exception is that the rule of unconditional help is superseded by a calculated give and take when care relationships are overriden by another set of relationships, not directly relevant to the Centre world. Thus, a few participants who were all in the process of leaving the Centre developed a strong mutual interest, and gave each other advice and help on matters concerning their future. Although elements deriving from the Centre reality were present in the relationship, matters such as plans for jobs and accommodation, and the resumption of family contacts were the dominant factors. This preoccupation precluded the group from taking an active part in the care system and created an internal pattern of care relationship, based on premeditated exchanges which did not allow one member to take advantage of the others without reciprocating almost immediately (see 'Differentiation').

The exclusion of mutuality in the rendering of help is most striking in situations of one-sided and recurrent care. Thus participants who help certain other participants on a fairly regular basis, assisting somebody to get downstairs, attending at the toilet, or pushing a wheelchair in and out of the Centre, do not expect and, indeed, do not usually receive any service or explicit reward in return. Invariably such relationships are taken as a matter of course, with neither the helpers nor the helped commenting on them.

Participants volunteer general statements on the value of care and the need to help, but refrain from mentioning individuals as targets for care. When participants deviate from this rule and disclose their beneficiaries, they usually face tacit disapproval, expressed mainly by silence.

This anonymity is significant for the development of impersonal channels of care, of which the most popular were the frequent sales held in the Centre, most of the goods being donated by participants. Another general, non-individual benefit was offered by the entertainment group. This was formed by two participants whose intention was 'to distribute happiness between people and to help them forget their troubles'. This was to be achieved by staging a light-hearted show of old-time songs and sketches.

The cast was to consist of seven participants and the relationship between them signified the predominance of the care norm over unevenly distributed artistic qualities. Thus, the pianist, who was a hard-of-hearing, retired dance musician, was helped to restore some of the standards of his heyday by incessant, tedious rehearsals with the rest of the cast. Replacements were available, but were not considered. A member of the cast who was critical of the pianist's accompaniment was told by the organizers to quit as 'we can not tolerate such an insult to a friend who has got to face such difficulties'. One of the singers was urged to take part in the concert 'because she is lonely and miserable and a bit of singing will do her good'. Another was recruited, despite his obvious inability to sing in tune, because 'It will be a good outlet for him after all the aggravation he has had with his family.'

When the concert party started its rounds of old age homes and day centres, an opportunity was given to participants who were not members of the cast to join the group and to boost response amongst the audience and thereby to share in the care situation created by the group.

Although the principle of boundless unconditional help impregnates the conduct of care relationships in the Centre, there are a few recognized limitations which circumscribe its operation. These arise from factors not germane to the care system, or from incongruities and contradictions in the system itself.

The first category includes exogenous limitations on participants' ability to help. Ill health was the major impediment, and participants frequently expressed frustration at being unable to help on account of their disabilities. As most of the participants suffered from some sort of handicap, situations such as helplessness in the face of an overturned wheelchair were not unusual. Another frustration occurred when participants were in excessive demand for help, and had to decline requests because of shortage of time. Nevertheless such participants were offended if the request to help was not made at all. One busy participant explained: 'At least I could have given them some advice on how to do it if I can't do it myself.'

Obstacles were also raised by outsiders. Thus, a request by participants to give a hand in dishing up and cleaning at the Jewish Blind Society's Centre was rejected by the supervisor of the place. Clubs and other day care establishments in the area also turned down overtures from participants.

Apparent failures in helping people overcome emotional distress were also a major source of frustration. A participant who was invited to officiate in a *seder* in an old age home described the experience as 'a bitter feeling of helplessness, not being able to do a thing to cheer these people up a bit'. In cases of bereavement attempts were always made to alleviate the grief, but often with no immediate effect.

Participants who, for one reason or another, refuse help, present another dimension to this problem. By denying other participants the right to help, the supremacy of care is put in question. Those rebuffed are put in an awkward position. They may rationalize the rejection or discredit the people who reject them.

Joseph (see 'The idea of care') as a homeless, lonely and poor participant was an obvious object for help and assistance was offered to him by a few participants who wished to clothe and accommodate him. Joseph rejected all these attempts, saying that the time had not yet arrived for his mission to be accomplished. Some participants accepted this retort and did not bother him again, but it nevertheless was beyond the comprehension of most members, who accused Joseph of being 'unreasonable', 'arrogant' and, therefore 'undeserving'.

Stanley, a participant with a long history of mental illness, who vacillated between different religious convictions and eventually became an extremely orthodox Jew, led many participants to question his emotional stability after he had refused to be helped in any way by any of them. Even seemingly insignificant gestures such as handing to him an ashtray, or offering to instruct him in his craftwork, were turned away. He isolated himself completely from the rest of the participants who regarded him as a 'maniac', 'lunatic', etc.

A different problem was presented by participants who were well integrated into the Centre life and helped other people, but while accepting help in some areas, refused to be looked after in others. Most of them were disabled participants who insisted on a high degree of independence. Some were also anxious to prove to themselves and to others that they were fully capable of performing ordinary acts, such as opening a door, or walking unaided, by displaying these abilities in front of others. Any attempt to give a hand was regarded as implying lack of confidence, and consequently this sort of help was invariably refused. Rejections of this sort were usually accepted as legitimate and understandable, as they could be construed within the context of the care system.

Able-bodied participants presented a more serious problem. They were fit enough to do an outside job, thus contradicting the view that only people who could not fend for themselves were entitled to Centre services. Some able-bodied participants, who did not take a great part in Centre life, and who regarded it as a sanctuary during a transitional period of hardship, were called 'parasites', 'extortionists', etc. An able-bodied participant, who did involve himself with the Centre reality, and was one of the stalwarts of the care system, could still find himself in embarrassing situations. After a discussion group he helped to remove some of the chairs from the room and unthinkingly hung three chairs on his arm and lifted them up. The others in the room thought this demonstration of physical prowess out of place, and offensive to the rest, who were not as fit as he was. Caustic, loud remarks, such as 'what is he doing in the Centre anyway?', or, 'he can easily earn his living as a docker', were heard. The man returned the chairs and carried on taking them out one by one.

Married couples, very good friends, in one case the fact that a mother and her son were both participants, contradicted by their close contact two principles of the care system. Care and help should be the predominant ingredient of relationships between people, and in each of those cases they composed only one aspect of a complex affiliation. Further, there was a strong element of mutuality between the partners in each case. They did not distribute their concern and resources indiscriminately amongst needy participants, but rather concentrated on their small, exclusive unit. This aroused a certain amount of antagonism and some of these couples were faced with isolation and disregard. Thus, in a fire drill held in the Jewish Blind Society centre the participants helped one another to get downstairs, but a disabled married couple was left unattended, deliberately overlooked by the rest. They had to make their own way down, with great difficulty.

Couples were often accused of excessive possessiveness, of not letting their partners participate fully in Centre life. The existence of independent care units within the general framework of the care system was regarded as intolerable and destructive by most of the participants.

An indication of the failure of the system, in the form of people leaving the Centre, as a result of physical or mental deterioration, was the most ominous threat to the validity of care, and indeed to the goal of the system: the arrest of change. The reaction was to eject the afflicted individual from the system by ceasing to help him, thereby escaping responsibility for the deterioration and even denying former affiliation. Such disengagements happened mainly when a participant was on the verge of being transferred to residential care.

One of the most popular participants, having suffered a series of crippling heart-attacks, became a transport user, and his general dependence on outside services such as hospitals, home-help and nursing increased considerably. He could no longer negotiate the stairs and had to spend all day in the downstairs lounge. His active involvement with Centre life had to be severely curtailed. Gradually he lost touch with events, and his former friends who witnessed his deterioration do not seem to have tried to restore his involvement. Rather, some expressed the opinion that he should be attended to by his wife, who was not a participant, as 'we can not do anything for him and it is a wife's job to look after her husband'.

Another illustration concerns a woman who was about to be admitted into an old age home. On the day of the disclosure the woman asked a member of the committee to see her over the road on her way to the bus stop. Usually such a request would have been granted promptly and readily, but this time she was told, 'This is the job of the staff, go and ask them, I haven't got time.'

Although some efforts were made to render care beyond the Centre, people were careful to circumscribe their activities, to protect the integrity of the care system. The intrusion of other realities might threaten the cognitive control over time, and raise the possibility of admitting unarrested deterioration.

The Jewish Blind Society centre was an arena upon which limitations of involvement were imposed. The main dissatisfaction with the experiment was expressed by the blind people, who criticized the unwillingness of participants to mingle with them, and to participate in their specific activities. This was explicitly denied, and counter allegations were made along the same lines. Nevertheless in private encounters participants emphasized that, as Jonathan put it, 'It is no good mixing with the blind, they have got their own world and we have got ours. Let us not destroy each other's world.' Again, such a response recalls characteristics of sectarian behaviour.

In the course of one of the discussions on old age homes, a few participants, who expressed willingness to go and help in such institutions, were warned by others that they would be in danger of 'vegetating' and 'becoming an inmate yourself'. Some withdrew. Others said that they were well aware of this hazard, but would take due care to avoid such a fate.

The integrity of the system's boundaries was also respected by individual participants, who refused help from other participants in tackling problems arising from their outside difficulties. Thus, one participant refused to allow others to help him in moving into a new flat. Another rejected offers to visit him in his bedsitter during an illness. Participants rarely expect other participants to visit them in hospital, although staff visits are arranged.

Care, being a central value in a social code governing the rules and norms of the Centre life, is also treated as a major resource in moulding power relationships amongst participants and between participants and staff. The pivotal role of care was most apparent in the operation of the committee and its benevolent fund. The committee was designed to consist of participants who were able to look after others, and its main target was to institutionalize patterns of care and help already in existence in the Centre.

Members of staff asked participants to see committee members merely as helpers of the staff. They worked for the participants and, therefore, deserved co-operation, but it was stressed that membership of the committee did not entail any official authority, and that participants should avoid identifying committee tasks with staff jobs, either in the range of responsibility or in power. In staff meetings the supervisor often said that serving on the committee was a therapeutic activity for its members, and this was its main significance as far as the staff were concerned.

Members of the committee, however, saw their function in the Centre in an entirely different light. They were convinced that the Centre could be run perfectly smoothly under the full control of the participants, and that the presence of staff was merely a necessary evil. Some of them maintained that as they helped and cared as much as members of staff did, if not more, they should be awarded the same respect and authority by their fellow participants. This trend reached its climax when a proposal was put forward and accepted in one of the committee meetings that badges showing their names should be worn by the members on their lapels. This was followed by a motion claiming entitlement to a free cup of tea, as 'we help as much as staff and like them we must get free tea'. This motion was turned down by the new supervisor on the grounds that it might arouse the envy of other participants who also helped, but did not happen to be on the committee. He argued further that membership of the committee was voluntary and if they chose to act as members it was only for their own self-glorification.

Committee members commanded some resources which could be utilized in a power struggle with staff. For example, the withdrawal of help in supervising the lunch attendance and compiling the register would mean an extra burden for staff. Threats to take such action were often voiced, but never materialized, and in fact the staff came to rely increasingly on help from volunteers, and from participants who were not on the committee.

The main demand posed was that more notice be taken of participants' views, that they be given more say in decision-making. This issue came to a head when the new supervisor took office. Having realized the utility of constructive co-operation with the committee, he promised to recognize their special status in the Centre but stressed that 'I am the boss here and I am going to run this place and if necessary dispense with the Committee.'

As members of the committee realized that anybody could perform their non-specialized, unskilled tasks, they tended to be cautious in their attempts to control participants. Thus when a quiz was prepared by a member of the committee, other participants were called 'to help' him to hold it and not just to attend it. Participation in other activities was also labelled 'help to help', as if this terminology was a diminutive form of asserting power and authority.

Nevertheless, critics drew a distinction between the sheer pursuit of power and genuine help. These sentiments were voiced mainly in general meetings, and caused arguments. A typical criticism was, 'There are some members of the Committee who really like to help and I have got nothing against them, but others are just power mad and they should be exposed.' The distinction between 'help' and 'power' was an issue in many committee meetings, notably when the organization of outings for participants was under discussion. The 'benevolent fund' sponsored transport and refreshments for days out and, although such undertakings were always made in close conjunction with staff, the financial onus of the enterprise was on the committee. Being responsible for such events entailed handling money, making decisions concerning places to visit, entertainment and recreations for the day. In effect, organizing an outing meant a temporary share in the actual control of the participants.

Following a suggestion from the new supervisor, a permanent sub-committee for organizing outings was elected. This brought to a head a long-standing rift between two factions of members inside the committee. The first, whose leader was elected as chairman of the new sub-committee, consisted of three participants who advocated closer co-operation with staff and the confinement of committee activities to an agreed area of entertainment and special events. The hard core of the second faction included two participants who conducted a not unsuccessful campaign over the daily running of the Centre. They demanded active participation in staff meetings and increased involvement in decision-making processes.

Having been elected, the leader of the 'conservative' faction consented to act as chairman only if people who were identified with the 'radical' clique were precluded from membership of his sub-committee. This condition was strongly opposed by most members and he was called upon to retract and apologize. Before he could react a full-scale row had erupted. Members accused each other of not being helpful enough, of neglecting their duties and the needs of the participants and, the gravest indictment of all, of being obsessed with power and not with genuine concern for the participants' welfare.

The 'conservatives' were condemned for pursuing personal goals outside the Centre rather than helping participants, while the 'radicals' were alleged to have introduced an authoritarian, hierarchical dimension into the relationship amongst participants. Both accusations were meant to expose deviations from the only legitimate form of care, which is help for the sake of help, with no immediate perks or expected future rewards.

The row, which reached a high pitch, was cooled down by the new supervisor, who threatened to disband the committee and even to resign. The apology demanded by the chairman was given, and the rivals decided that there was so much to do in the Centre that there was ample room for the co-existence of different groups of helpers and of complementary methods of help.

The care system and the organization of time

The lack of any apparent direct form of exchange is perhaps the most striking aspect of the care system. The emphasis is on the relationship between a participant and the overall system. Although participants are continuously involved in face-to-face interaction, there is an evident element of impersonal relationships.

People are related to each other by virtue of their commitment to the idea of care, rather than by the attributes of their specific personalities and interests. This is relevant to the social construction of time.

Mauss (1954, p.34) phrased the association between exchange and time as follows:

> In any society it is in the nature of the gift in the end to be its own reward. By definition, a common meal, a distribution of *kava*, or a charm worn, cannot be repaid at once. Time has to pass before counter presentation can be made. Thus, the notion of time is logically implied when one pays a visit, contracts a marriage or an alliance, makes a treat, goes to organized games, fights or feasts of others, renders rituals and honorific services and shows respect.

Or, in Titmuss's words (1973, p.82), 'the notion of time in relation to acts of giving and receiving is significant and implies the further notion of credit.'

The social reality in the Centre lacks the element of 'credit', of anticipation of a like return. Therefore, the intrinsic notion of time must be rather different from the one distilled in the exchange relationships described by Mauss. Giving or receiving are completely divorced from calculations of cost, or prospective gains or profits. However, the lack of predictability and planning does not necessarily mean insecurity, for participants can be reasonably sure, within the limitations described, that care and concern will be rendered to them regardless of their personal balance of past investment and future potentialities. The knowledge that compliance with the code of behaviour embedded in the care system provides relative security within the Centre environment, whilst imposing no demands to fulfil any specific obligations, engenders a new conception of the relation between events. Participants may perceive actions by themselves or by fellow participants as not necessarily affecting each other. Such a conception excludes a time perspective which sees the past causing the future. The present itself contains only the actual engagement of the moment.

The Centre routine presented a potential threat to this construction of time. Making the Centre a staff-free territory was an essential prerequisite if the organization of activities by participants was to correspond to their conception of the relations between events.

An attempt to follow the daily routine of the Centre reveals a lack of progressive continuity between events. As in giving and taking, one event is not necessarily linked to the other in terms of actual planning and anticipation. Hypothetically at least, one could easily reorder and rearrange events without any discernible effect.

The discussion on the routine in the Centre has already raised a number of points relevant to this issue. There are no precise expectations that participants will act and do things along certain lines, they enjoy relative autonomy, including the freedom to walk in and out whenever they like, and to refuse to commit themselves to a defined pattern of participation. Wide leeway is left for participants to negotiate transport and lunch arrangements, and they are free to form their own groups and to organize activities independent of staff. All in all, an arena is constructed in which a scheduled, premeditated routine is liable to be constantly subjected to uncertainties and last-minute alterations.

The content of the activities is as important as the structure in defining relations between events. A comprehensive, widely used term in the Centre to describe the perceived effect of the range of activities held there is 'atmosphere'. Participants and staff alike talked of a 'good atmosphere', a 'friendly atmosphere', a 'cordial/convivial/frivolous/light-hearted atmosphere', etc.

A typical afternoon in the Centre begins with a talk given by an outsider, normally introduced by a member of staff. This is followed by a short discussion. The rest of the afternoon is composed of a jumble of simultaneous activities, indistinguishable from one another and engrossing all the participants. The amplification system is switched on and the microphone is used freely and in a disorderly fashion by participants to sing, tell jokes, and to have a chat with the audience. This invariably leads to a 'singsong', accompanied by piano playing and old gramophone records. Participants who do not take part in the musical entertainment are engaged in small talk, and card games, and sometimes raffles and bingo games are spontaneously organized. The afternoon ends with shifting the tables and chairs to one side to clear a space for an 'old time dance'. Attempts to introduce some order into the seeming disorder by laying down a timetable, allocating different entertainment roles amongst participants, and regulating the use of the microphone, were completely disregarded.

Most of these activities are also held on Sunday afternoons, and had it been up to the participants, they would have been extended to fill the whole week. Each of these activities deserves detailed account and analysis, but my immediate concern is with their repetitive nature. Not only the type and general outlines of an activity are repeated, but also the content. The same jokes are told endlessly, and the same songs, accompanied by the same gestures and mannerisms, are sung time and time again.

The songs and dances represent à rather limited selection of music hall and variety entertainment of the late 1920s and early 1930s, with improvisations and additions. Attempts to introduce different types of entertainment into this framework, such as classical and cantoral music, or even 'pop' records, produced no response. The idea of the Centre as a 'Darby and Joan' club was widely accepted and encouraged by participants, who found the analogy with a cabaret or music hall apt. Famous music hall entertainers were frequently mentioned and mimed, and their life histories and shows were the subject of daily conversations, quizzes and arguments.

Card games and bingo contribute a complementary facet to the repetitious and seemingly aimless recreation in the Centre. As the sums of money involved are of no material importance, the pay-off comes in the very act of performing them repetitively and with a high degree of engrossment. In this way they smoothly fit into the other activities of the same nature. In contrast to Goffman's analysis of games (1972), there are very few rules of irrelevance to delineate the boundaries between playing and engaging in 'serious' social encounters. In a sense, one can question the very definition of such activities as 'games', as their integration in the overall social context of the Centre does not distinguish them from any other facet of the Centre reality.

It seems significant that card players were reprimanded for continuing the game only when the Centre reality was being threatened by outside elements. Thus whenever religion or old age homes were discussed, participants who continued playing were criticized. In some instances, physical force was used to stop them playing.

Innovation and creativity were systematically stifled. Social workers in the Centre regularly complained about the apathy shown to proposals for new activities requiring initiative and programming. A suggestion to set up art-appreciation classes was rejected out of hand as 'a laugh', and when a sketching group was eventually formed, its members demanded detailed instructions and guidance in their work. Similarly, craft work done by participants invariably followed conventional designs in a limited range of articles, mainly mosaic-coated ashtrays, simple toys, and raffia work. A participant who decided to go to council art classes in the evenings and to practise his studies in the Centre, using imaginative and original designs and ideas, was ridiculed, and no other participants followed suit. Although he was encouraged and held up as an example by staff, he became more and more isolated and eventually found that even the few participants who had taken an interest in talking to him preferred to disengage themselves from his company.

The unwillingness of participants to show initiative, display individuality or to depart from the norms penetrated almost every aspect of the activities. A 'talent competition' held by a member of staff received such a poor response that the only contender was the member of staff, who awarded himself the first prize. It proved impossible to get participants to contribute original material to the Centre magazine, *News and Views*. The paper was mostly composed of trite jokes, well-known songs and poems, and pieces of information about past Centre activities. The very few short stories or essays written by participants seemed to be an unwelcome appendix to the rest.

Two events which contained potential for planning and progress were converted into care situations where the element of advancement was completely overshadowed by the predominance of the care system. The first was a drama group set up by a social worker who claimed that his 'creativity and unusual ideas' failed to gain the co-operation of participants. The group was meant to put on a reading performance of Arnold Wesker's play *Chicken Soup with Barley*, which concerns life in the East End, covering places, events and characters well-known to most of the participants. The idea was that it would offer ground for identification, and so an opportunity for participants to express themselves, and to stage a reflection of their own life histories.

After an arduous search for a cast, the group was formed and rehearsals took place. It would be unfair to judge the dramatic qualities of an amateur group in this context, but an impression of lack of enthusiasm and interest was inescapable. The only revival of the rehearsals occurred when members of the cast talked about their difficulties in following and reading aloud the text because of poor eyesight, a bad throat or other physical impediments. Such complaints provoked immediate offers of help and advice, and cast members who seemed to have achieved some degree of improvement were applauded and encouraged to continue. It emerged that the main target of the group was not putting on the play, but using the rehearsals as another care situation.

This became evident when the director – the social worker – decided the time had come to stage the show in front of the participants and a few invited guests from the Board. The reaction was less than lukewarm. The cast postponed the date for the show and eventually deferred it indefinitely. When the social worker in charge had to go away for a few weeks the rehearsals were not held and when discord arose over the reluctance of the cast to go and see a professional performance of the play, the group dispersed and the whole idea of a show by participants died out.

The concert party group revitalized the idea of a show by participants for participants with much more success. A group was formed which aimed 'to distribute happiness amongst participants and to cheer them up'. From the first rehearsal the group acted as a care environment for its members, who were judged and acclaimed not according to the merits of their performances, but on the basis of their willingness to help other members of the cast to overcome their difficulties. Attempts to excel as a performer or to introduce original material were persistently suppressed.

A member of the cast who claimed to be the star singer of the show and maintained that he had received invitations to appear in other day centres was ridiculed and his statements were dismissed as unfounded. Another cast member who contributed a song which he claimed was original was told that the song had been heard before on the radio and was by no means original. (As it happens the song, although containing some trite themes borrowed from popular tunes, apparently was written by the participant.) A request to the organizer to include some pieces written by participants was turned down on the grounds that 'they might be too subtle and we need only well-known stuff which people can immediately recognize and have a good laugh'. Thus, the end product was, to the evident enjoyment of the audience, a show not very different from the daily afternoon 'sing songs'.

The care system thus generates a framework for acts and events in which no element of progression, planning or order is discernible. Yet the Centre does not seem chaotic. The relation between the various elements in its social reality are determined by the accepted code of attitudes and behaviour which imply an overall conception of time and care.

The care relationship and the organization of activities in the Centre may be seen as a system of re-integration, eliminating the incongruities of the limbo state and permitting the development of a coherent conception of the later phase of the life cycle. It displaces the frustrating, unattainable targets of progress, planning, materialistic and social achievements in favour of a contrasting yet orderly and organized framework for establishing relationships and views. Thus, instead of limited resources distributed, allocated and accumulated on the basis of a zero-sum conception of the social situation, there is only one, unlimited resource, allocated on the assumption of a non-zero-sum world. The exclusion of reciprocity from the care relationship makes each act of help a unique enterprise unrelated to obligations, and as such bearing special merit. In Simmel's words (1964, p.392), 'Once we have received something good from another person, once he has preceded us with his action we can no longer make up for it completely, no matter how much our own return gift or service may objectively or legally surpass his own.'

Barriers of hierarchy, power, stratification and status are smoothed out by the unlimited availability of the care resource. At the same time, the boundaries between the system and the outside world are rigidly delineated. The demand for full commitment to the Centre code of care relationship, plus disengagement from the outside world, creates a situation in which the Centre world becomes a plausible alternative reality.

5   The limbo society

The community of participants faces various problems in effecting the transformation of a time-bound elderly person. Moreover, the society of participants into which a newcomer is drawn, although based on the principles of the care system, is composed of various groups and categories. The following sections examine these issues. They are followed by an analysis of the ways and means used by participants to control their social world, and to guard the care system from potentially destructive elements.

Initiation

It is not altogether misleading to speak of 'initiation' into the Centre. There is the basic fact of segregation from society. The participants are excluded from the outside world of stratification and mobilization, and secluded within an enclave. Here they renounce elements of their past, obliterate differentiations, and create a common denominator founded on the ideas of equality and fraternity. The manipulation of the care concept makes of the Centre environment an alternative reality, in which the individual can construct a new social world for himself.[1]

Nevertheless, the analogy should not be pressed too far. In the Centre itself, there is no element of transition from one reality to another, nor is there any continuity linking it to an outside reality. There is no element of preparing the participants to enter a new phase in their lives, nor is there any attempt to transform the Centre into a different environment from what it is. Although there are some traces of millenarian or apocalyptic notions in some participants' worldviews, they are by no means predominant features of the Centre reality. There are no official instructors, no official novices, no recognized stages through which participants pass, and no social recognition of the conversion.[2]

Yet newcomers do undergo certain fundamental changes in their outlook on life and their conception of social relationships. On numerous occasions participants expressed the immense impact of the Centre on their lives, and the complete alteration of character involved in joining the Centre. The main trend of transformation seemed to follow a common pattern. Participants described their pre-Centre situations as 'vegetating', 'being a cabbage', and 'death so to speak', whereas attendance was alleged to endow them with 'a new lease of life', 'new spirit' and almost invariably a feeling of happiness and fulfilment.

Most of the participants who claimed to have undergone the transformation stated that initially they came to the Centre for the material advantages it offered. However, in no time, this view of the Centre as a convenient and cheap communal kitchen was replaced by total submersion in the new reality. This process can be analysed into various elements and stages.

Perhaps the most striking encounter with the new environment is the adjustment to changes in the manner of personal address and reference. There is extensive use of first names, or avoidance of names instead of surnames preceded by the prefix, Mr, Miss or Mrs. Participants who had known each other for a long time, maintained stable ongoing relationships and took part in the same activities, were often ignorant of the full names of their partners. Others just used nicknames or abbreviated names to address a particular participant, or in referring to him.

The participant whose duty it was to compile the daily register of attendance was confronted with a number of members who just walked past him without giving their names. Some simply expected him to recall their names. Those who did co-operate usually gave their forenames or their Centre nicknames. Joseph, reflecting on the scenes this provoked (mostly angry arguments between the registrar and an offended participant whose name had slipped his memory), once said: 'This is very similar to what happens in primitive tribes and some religious sects when people are given new names.' This insight certainly did apply to a few participants who actually altered their names. The following social worker's report on a participant may illustrate such a process:

(Upon first attendance): 'Although it is nine months since his wife passed away he is still grieving and broke down during my interview. He is having difficulty in adjusting to his new situation and gets very depressed. He cannot get himself to go out to clubs and other social activities. He cannot manage his finance.'

After two years these 'negative' traits have on the whole disappeared:

'Still grieving deeply the loss of his wife. Is not interested in clubs. Happy at home. Changed his name ... because "people cannot remember his name". His behaviour in the Centre now is far from appearing depressed and weak kneed, he is very much on the make expressing uncautiously his moans and groans to staff and participants alike. He is very anxious not to be undone....

He becomes one of the Centre's stalwarts.

The comments made in my previous report are not now relevant....

His spirit remains high and there is official talk of his getting married again.'

The correlation between the change of name and transition from a state of bereavement and grief indicates the final stage of initiation. The initial phase is, however, filled with confusion, vacillation and perplexity. Here other participants play a major part in preparing the novice for the inculcation of the code of the care system. At this initial stage there are two major issues: the reaction of participants to the problems of encountering a recent loss suffered by the newcomer; and the way in which the newcomer puts together the elements necessary to becoming a 'centre-centred' participant.

Grief is treated in a seemingly ambivalent way. On the one hand participants are very determined to ignore the subject of death and seldom make reference to the deceased (see 'The ultimate reality'). On the other hand, attempts to console and alleviate grief constitute an integral part of the care system. Bereaved participants were not reminded of their grief unless they themselves broached the subject. In that event they were usually given a sympathetic hearing and advised to try and forget the past, and to consider the recovery other participants had made after experiencing a similar calamity. The main line taken in such cases was that there is nothing unusual in losing a spouse and that most members of the Centre had shared the same experience, overcome the blow and adjusted themselves to a happy active existence in the Centre.

But newcomers are made to realize that communicating their personal problems produces no positive reactions – at best a polite platitude, and at worst complete disregard. Instead they can arouse interest and concern by discussing experiences in hospitals, or by asking for help and advice on matters concerning health and social services. Newcomers are quick to learn that complaining about physical disabilities makes no impact unless accompanied by a request for help. They are also helped to adjust to the Centre's timetable, activities, physical structure and institutions (e.g. committee, benevolent fund). Instructions on these vital matters are given meticulously and promptly, without the newcomer even asking for them.

All newcomers experience the same general phase of introduction into Centre life. The process of initiation, however, takes various courses, and individuals experience different stages. Instead of generalizing, therefore, I shall discuss a few cases ranging from instances of successful integration into the Centre to instances in which participants failed to assimilate.

Case 1

Judith – a newcomer suffering from severe emotional distress after losing her son in a road accident – made her first approach in the Centre to a member of staff who referred her to Lewis and Jack, two members of the committee who were known for the avid interest they took in looking after newcomers. They welcomed her and suggested that however deep her sorrow might have been, she should try and forget it by mingling with 'the happy family of the Centre'.

Judith was evidently moved by this welcome, and said that she would try to co-operate and mingle with Lewis's friends. Later she privately made it clear to me that she had made up her mind to help Lewis as 'he seems to be a very brave man who manages to stay happy despite his disabilities'. In the following weeks Judith made more and more acquaintances and formulated her intention to do everything in her power to look after other participants less fortunate than herself. She claimed that having seen so much misery and anguish amongst participants, she had undergone a reassessment of her attitude towards her own problems. The

Centre, therefore, had completely changed her outlook on life, which was henceforth to be devoted to helping other people. She even talked about working in a voluntary capacity in a hospital for the incurable.

Case 2

Whereas Judith was a 'successful convert' from the beginning of her participation, Alfred did not respond to advances made to him by Lewis and Jack and, although able-bodied, preferred to stay inert in the lounge, seemingly withdrawn into himself. Lewis gave up any hope of involving Alfred in the Centre life, and attributed the failure to his being 'simple'. Lewis's wife, however, maintained that this was a false impression and that perseverance would produce results. She tried to persuade Alfred to do some craft work or to talk about his problems, but to no avail. Nevertheless, when she asked for his help in doing the washing-up after tea he did not refuse and even took the opportunity to ask her advice on treatment for his rheumatism. This marked the beginning of Alfred's active involvement in the Centre. He took craftwork instruction from Lewis and his wife, helped in serving the tea, and participated in discussion groups. He also received a secondhand transistor radio from one of the participants ('my only entertainment in my bedsitter'), and a ticket to a musical from another. Gradually he extended his scope by assisting the disabled, moving furniture and running errands. The change in his spirit was remarkable. He said he only started living in the Centre.

Case 3

Like Alfred, Saul was admitted into the Centre following the death of his wife. However, he was also afflicted by a rapid deterioration of his hearing. This was particularly unbearable since he was a music lover, and had earned his living as a professional dance pianist. As Saul put it, 'I don't know what was worse, losing my wife or losing my hearing. If I had to choose I would have chosen for the first to happen.' Indeed, in his first days at the Centre he found nothing to talk about but his hearing aid, but as many other participants had similar appliances, a wide area for initial communication was created.

When the concert party entertainment group was formed Saul was invited to be the pianist. The first rehearsals showed he was completely out of tune, and it was obvious that the standard of his playing was far from satisfactory even for an amateur performance. Nevertheless, the members of the group were determined 'to make a go of it' and not to let Saul down. Hence, they spent hours in the Centre rehearsing each note with him until he achieved an acceptable degree of harmony with the cast. The fact that Saul was hard of hearing was announced to the audience on the night of the show and his solo performance won special applause. Members of the cast who criticized his playing were expelled from the group for 'not trying to help'. An offer made by the new supervisor's wife to become the group's pianist, after she had occasion temporarily to replace Saul, was rejected. Saul continued to make appearances with the group in their 'happiness distribution' tour of old age homes and day centres. Alongside this major activity, he also took part in the daily life of the Centre and from being a meek, subdued participant he changed into an outgoing and talkative personality, disregarding his hearing difficulties and helping other participants.

Novices who hold to strong personal convictions and beliefs contradictory to some of the teachings of the Centre, may cause discord and opposition, but they do not face isolation and ostracism as long as they comply with the main principles of the care system.

Cases 4 and 5

Two newcomers accepted these basic principles although one still adhered to his preoccupation with politics and the other persisted in discussing religion. (Both had renounced their families.) They argued continually, each insisting on bringing up his favourite subject unless the other would drop his. This was kept up for a few months until the rest of the participants made it clear that neither would be heard unless they dropped the two taboo topics. They accepted this, and the two became the guardians of the rule forbidding the introduction of either politics or religion.

Direct social pressure was rarely exerted to enforce conversion, and in the few cases in which sanctions were imposed they were unsuccessful. It is impossible to define the exact factor determining assimilation into the Centre or the rejection of its world. Nevertheless, there are indications that the critical point should be sought in the occasional incompatibility between certain elements in the Centre's code of principles and personal idiosyncrasies. A few cases of unsuccessful adjustment will be examined in an attempt to ascertain the role personality plays in the course of initiation.

The inhibition of shame and indignity associated with entering the Centre can present an insuperable barrier to a newcomer with ongoing affiliations outside. An extended illustration of such a case will be given later (see 'Differentation'), but this was not an isolated one.

Case 6

A local politician who was also an active representative in the British Zionist Federation had to attend the Centre following the death of his wife and a severe illness. He hardly responded to approaches made to him by other participants, and was mainly interested in showing-off papers confirming his association with Jewish political organizations and community institutions, matters which interested nobody else in the Centre. His condescension towards other participants and his outside concerns prevented his inclusion in Centre activities.

Participants suffering from mental disorders were invariably treated as ordinary members regardless of their disability. Symptoms indicating psychological problems were mostly regarded as a reaction to environmental factors, such as isolation and alienation rather than to an inherent instability, and therefore participants normally expect a change in the behaviour and spirit of such people after exposure to the Centre surroundings. In most cases of depression the improvement was indeed remarkable, and it is reasonable that in the absence of medical knowledge and information about the mental state of a participant, a similar course of recovery would be generally anticipated. The following case will demonstrate what happens when such a theory fails.

Case 7

Sid was a manic-depressive who suffered a severe relapse following a car crash involving his son. He arrived at the Centre subdued, withdrawn and completely unresponsive. Attended by his wife, who acted as a volunteer in the Centre, he withdrew to a corner and spent his days gazing blankly at the others. A sudden change in his condition reversed the whole situation. Sid entered into a state of boundless elation and exhilaration, became extremely talkative and active, declared his intention to take part in all Centre activities and offered to help far beyond his capabilities. This transformation was welcomed by participants as a response to their incessant efforts and to the influence of the Centre atmosphere. Sid was introduced to outsiders as the 'great success', 'miraculous recovery', etc., statements which were invariably echoed by Sid himself, who would reassure the listener that he felt fine and that his only concern was to look after people who might have been through similar emotional distress. In discussion groups and informal gatherings, Sid always brought up the subject of helping other participants and preached the teachings of the care system to whoever was ready to listen.

Petty bickerings and brawls with participants, coupled with unfounded claims to membership of the committee and to power 'officially' delegated to him by staff, provided the first indications that Sid was diverting from the expected path of initiation, and might even prove to be a menace, particularly to the care system. In fact, occasional bouts of depression and recurrent defiance made it virtually impossible to handle Sid within the care system rules. The reaction amongst participants was to convert Sid into the Centre jester – a figure to be ridiculed, not to be taken seriously and yet to be integrated into the light-hearted, joking, atmosphere of the Centre. Thus, everything Sid said, regardless of its logical merits and contextual relevance, aroused laughter. His mere presence seemed to provoke waves of gaiety, and his apparent co-operation in building up this image contributed to establish this status. Gradually Sid sank into a long spell of depression and withdrew completely from the Centre activities. Only then was he recognized by his fellow participants as 'mental', 'sick' and 'a psychiatric case'.

Turning Sid into a clown was a measure taken by participants to tackle an ambiguous conversion – too good at the beginning and self-contradictory later on – although the convert himself did not question the intensity of his participation. In other cases, however, the decision to discontinue initiation is often made by the newcomer, and in more than one instance first encounters with the

Centre were such a shattering experience that attendance was discontinued. An example of this was given in the supervisor's first report on the Centre:[3]

> 'Several applicants have not been attracted to the Centre although they have attended. Obviously it is up to the social worker to ascertain the degree of motivation and if necessary to support clients in the first instance. As with initial interviews their first impression of the Centre can be all important. A recent example can illustrate this: a youthful-seeming applicant of 59 with a chronic heart condition was asked to attend the Centre without the direct support of the sponsoring social worker. His first impression was of the coach which picks up disabled people. As all of these participants were considerably older, both in appearance and attitudes than this gentleman – an impression confirmed when he actually saw participants in action at the Centre, he felt insulted that the Board had found fit to categorize him with "old fogies".'

Case 8

One evening, just before the last group of participants was about to leave, a confused-looking, slovenly-dressed man, accompanied by a well-known community do-gooder, entered the premises and asked for a social worker. None was immediately available and a conversation began with a few participants. The newcomers introduced themselves as Mark and Levy. They explained that they had come because Mark suffered from agoraphobia. Mark himself started listing his illnesses, medications and personal troubles, but was cut short by Lewis. 'Leave it mate, we all here have troubles of our own. Here in the Centre we don't talk about them, we try to forget.' This statement was echoed by other participants who added that if Mark did join the Centre they would help him as much as they could. One of them offered to instruct Mark for the first few days, guiding him in timetables and Centre regulations. He concentrated particularly on lunch procedures, and insisted that Mark should sit by him and follow his example.

Mark did not seem to be completely satisfied with the offer of help and readiness to accept him. His main concern was with the compulsory side of the craft work done in the Centre. 'I want to know where the factory is and how many hours a day I have to work there.' His fears were alleviated instantly. He was told that no obligations to work would be imposed on him and that everybody enjoyed the choice not to work. However, Mark still appeared to be discontented and asked whether anybody was interested in classical music or in languages. This query was disregarded.

Despite his evident qualms, Mark promised to come again the following morning, 'but not to eat, just to look around'. He emphasized that only when he had decided to settle as a participant would he cancel the daily 'meals on wheels' deliveries he was receiving. The following day Mark wandered around the Centre trying to no avail to initiate conversations on classical music and languages. Towards lunch time Mark decided to go home and was never seen again in the Centre.

This case draws attention to the critical relationship between the instructor and the novice. Although there is no set of rules to govern the interaction, certain parameters are clear. The extremes of remoteness and over-involvement leave no leeway for the instructor to operate. There must be some hope of changing and converting a novice.

Case 9

A married couple arrived at the Centre and, not having been introduced to anybody, chose to sit at a corner table, remote but not out of sight of the rest of the participants. Their youngish, well-groomed appearance together with the fact that they were not engaged in any work made them appear out of place. Participants who tried to approach them received polite answers but no encouragement. One of the participants demanded that the committee should handle them as 'they are not working-class people, the Centre is not a place for them'. A member of the committee tried to make a fresh start with the couple, but by then they seemed to be so shattered and confused that they failed to respond. This was interpreted by some participants as a sign of a condescending attitude, which proved that the couple should not be regarded as suitable to attend the Centre. The agitated atmosphere calmed down when the shaken couple rose and left the Centre.

The underlying view that attendance is restricted by class-identification was seldom expressed by participants. Nevertheless class-consciousness should not be underestimated as one of the perceived latent criteria for distinguishing the Centre people from outsiders.

Case 10

The opposite extreme of over-enthusiastic involvement is represented by the case of Ben who on first attendance proclaimed that the Centre was 'a wonderful, friendly place', the participants 'nice people', the lunches 'excellent' and that he could not have been happier. The participants who surrounded Ben looked at him with bewildered astonishment, and a few of them even pointed a finger to their heads, implying some uncertainty as to Ben's mental stability. Thenceforth no further attempt was made to communicate with him.

Differentiations

Equalizing extrinsic differences, suppressing quirks and idiosyncracies and insisting on an egalitarian code does not necessarily produce an 'egalitarian' society. There are within the Centre distinctive categories and groups.

The distinction participants draw between the 'able-bodied' and 'disabled' is not really based on an objective grading according to fitness. Three overlapping oppositions are invoked in making the distinction: (a) between people who attend the first or second of the two lunch sittings, (b) between 'transport people' and those not in need of this service, and (c) between the participants who spend their day in the downstairs lounge and those who attend the upstairs hall.

Each category includes a few people who might have chosen to join the other set. In particular, attendance at the first sitting rather than the second session for lunch is a matter of choice for people who do not require transport. Similarly, a number of participants marooned in their armchairs in the downstairs lounge are perfectly capable of making their way to the upstairs hall. A few of the 'transport people', although severely handicapped, manage to negotiate the stairs and to sit amongst the bulk of the able-bodied participants upstairs – and for the most part they are not classified as disabled within the Centre. Thus, the distinction is based on selection of territories and resources. Identification with one category entails a host of social implications for relationships with staff and with the other category of participants.

The most obtrusive difference in the relationship with staff is the high extent of dependency that marks the disabled as opposed to the relative physical autonomy enjoyed by the able-bodied. Transport is perhaps the main arena for displaying the inability of the handicapped to look after themselves, but having to be helped with lunches, moving about, communicating with other participants and, most important of all, being in constant need of the social worker's intervention in alleviating unbearable home situations and liaising with other agencies – mainly local authorities – all represent a very high degree of dependency. Attendance and flexibility of daily participation are regulated and monitored by staff and, therefore, the organization of time for the disabled cannot wholly emerge from the care-system principles. Able-bodied participants are in contrast less dependent and can sometimes afford to involve themselves in attempts to overrule staff decisions or, alternatively, cognitively to obliterate the existence of members of staff, so that the feeling of freedom and autonomy is complete and maintained.

The dependency of the disabled on staff represents a fundamental inconsistency in the care system. The principles of boundless and unconditional help seem to be incongruous with the sheer reality of participants being exclusively looked after by members of staff. The situation was well recognized by participants and staff alike and was considered to be a major point of tension between the two. Such discord emerged in committee meetings when participants accused members of staff of neglecting the disabled and directing too few resources towards their care. A few members maintained that as the Centre was partly supported by a local authority grant, allocated according to the number of registered disabled catered for by the establishment, it would be unfair to deprive the handicapped, who after all were supposed to be the beneficiaries of this money, of full participation in Centre activities. At the instance of a woman member of the committee, who was confined to a wheelchair, a resolution was passed that a special party for handicapped people be held in the Centre, hosted and prepared by the committee. The staff made no objection, and during the event able-bodied participants were strictly barred from the premises, admission being granted solely to voluntary helpers.

The success of the party stimulated an attempt to take over part of the transport operation. A decision by the committee to organize an outing for both disabled and able-bodied participants was over-ruled by the new supervisor, who maintained that the handicapped participants were the responsibility of the staff, and that the committee had neither adequate facilities nor the experience to look after disabled people. As the driver took orders only from the supervisor, the initiative seemed lost. A few committee members did suggest hiring coaches at the expense of the 'benevolent fund', but the supervisor warned the committee that if they went ahead 'I will call the police to prevent it and disperse the committee'.

The staff was united in resisting efforts by the committee to tres-pass on their authority by taking care of the disabled. The commit-tee was described as consisting of people who were 'power mad', 'full of self-importance', and 'inefficient'. The danger of a take-over attempt by the committee was seriously discussed in staff meetings, and by no means dismissed out of hand. It was evident that the staff viewed the issue as a power struggle, and were pre-pared to go a long way to fight it. The members, however, were particularly concerned to protect and extend their ideology of unlimited care, and considerations of power seemed less funda-mental.

The day following the supervisor's warning, two members of the committee spread the rumour that lunch time would be the zero hour for decisive action against the staff. Using expressions such as 'Here comes the revolution', and, 'We are going to show them', they managed to give the impression that a well-planned 'coup' was going to take place. As tension mounted and the second sitting was held, a presentation for a departing member of staff was made by the committee. It became clear that there would be no climax to the build-up, and the tension subsided into roars of laughter.

A few days later some members of the committee complained amongst themselves that most of the disabled participants would simply not accept any help and, therefore, that there was no sense in offering it, or in getting involved in arguments with staff over ways of entertaining them and including them in the Centre activi-ties. When later the idea of extending the Centre operation to late evenings and Sundays was broached, it was obvious that without a well-organized transport system the project would be bound to exclude the disabled. Nevertheless, when this drawback was mentioned a number of participants stressed that it was very

unlikely that the handicapped would want to attend, as they preferred their home environment to the Centre.

The balance between participation and commitment to out-
Centre life was also crucial to the second main opposition, between
men and women attending the Centre. This was significant. There
were gatherings consisting solely of women and others attended
only by men. The upper hall could easily be divided into two distinctive territories – one dominated by women doing needlework
and the other – well apart from them – inhabited by men doing
craftwork. There is one area in the middle, in which the two sexes
mingle occasionally. The same rule applies to the downstairs
lounge, where men tend to assemble in one corner whilst the
women gather in a separate row of chairs. Moreover, women pre-
dominate in keep-fit classes and in 'feminine' recreations such as
craft classes, beauty classes, etc., whereas the men are mostly
interested in discussion groups, talks and quizzes. Both sexes are
equally involved in the entertainment side of the Centre life.

Participants and staff alike were well aware of the distinction.
The line usually taken by participants was that 'we haven't got that
much in common.' Women led most of their lives in the family
circle and at home, whereas men went out to work, so there were
very few areas of shared interest. A number of male participants
maintained that most of the female participants still had attach-
ments to their families and homes which outweighed their commitment to the Centre. In support of this claim they used to point to
the absence of women on Fridays ('They have got to prepare for the
weekend'), and especially on the eves of Jewish festivals. In fact,
quite a few of the women in the Centre used the need to see to their
homes and cooking as an excuse for not attending occasionally.
Most of the men living on their own took advantage of jumble sales
and kitchenware sales, while the women kept themselves apart with
no evident signs of interest. The great bulk of the buyers of used
clothes and utensils were men and, had it not been for their interest,
the continuation of sales in the Centre would have been threatened.

It is evident that the main difference between men and women in
the Centre is rooted in their outside life. Some of the origins of the
distinction can be detected in the following piece, taken from the
participants' magazine:

THE PRIZE

About two months ago I read in the Woman's Page of the *Jewish Chronicle* that the editor of that page asked for letters from members, what they wanted from their Friendship Clubs and offered prizes of £1 each to the best ones. So I sent in mine and four or five weeks later, when I had almost forgotten about it, my husband, as usual, brought home the J.C. and after he had scanned the columns for Golden Weddings and Deaths (nisht du gaducht), handed it to me. I always look first on the back page to see the time Shabbos begins, and then at 'Woman's Page' now called 'You', and I saw my letter printed there. I gave a childish shriek (second childhood one) of delight and called out 'Sam, my letter is in the J.C.' He answered 'I didn't see it there.'

Well, it wasn't in the Deaths Column, thank God, and our own Golden Wedding was a year or so ago, so how could he. Be that as it may, several days ago, a letter and cheque for £1 arrived from the J.C. It was such a thrill. Anyone would think I had won the £25,000 premium Bond prize.

'Are you going to spend it or frame it?' asked my man.

Well, now I have a problem. With Chanuka drawing nigh and I always get a little something for each one of my family at that time, and as I splashed paint all over my overall, I need a new one. So any letters with suggestions in our *News and Views* will be welcomed, and the grand prize will be a 'Lolly Pop'. By the way, if you decide that I should spend my prize for Chanuka gifts, let me give you a list of recipients: 7 grandchildren, 1 great grandchild (aged 19 months) plus their parents. A 'layben' on them all.

My family always read *News and Views* so they know I am kidding.

Happy Chanuka to all!

This woman is still obviously attached to her family, her home chores and to some of the customs relating to Jewish festivals and traditions. She has plans, although 'mock' ones, and unlike her husband, is still clinging to the minute details of everyday life. The difference in perspectives is encapsulated in the difference of their reading habits.

Retirement, illness and bereavement had a much greater effect

on men than on women. The links with other environments were
abruptly severed and as the division of labour within the family
excluded the husband from taking an active part in the daily
running of the household, the new situation of living alone did not
offer any sense of continuation, and holding on to a well-controlled
environment, as in the case of most women. It is, therefore, hardly
surprising that involvement and assimilation into the Centre was
typically greater for men than women. This is strongly reflected in
the fact that the chief bearers of the care system – the participants
who formulated its principles, guarded its preservation and inculcated its values to newcomers – were mostly men.

Like the first opposition between the able-bodied and the
disabled, the distinction between men and women is based on the
balance between regarding the Centre reality as the core of one's
life and relying on other resources for care, interest and orientation.
The high dependency on staff by the handicapped contributed to
their separation from the rest of the participants, and the outward-
looking concerns of the women differentiated them from the men.

The extent of commitment constituted the major lines along
which groups were formed and disbanded. Groups of participants
may be identified according to conventional sociological criteria,
taking into account regularity of meetings, relatively stable
membership and shared activities. Using these criteria one might
delineate four distinctive groups.

The first centred around Jack and Lewis, who also led the
'radical' clique in the committee (see 'Patterns of help'). They both
maintained that the Centre is the only meaningful way of existence
they have experienced and, therefore, that there should be no limits
to devotion to it. Indeed the two of them spent most of their time in
the place, played a major role in organizing activities such as the
concert party tour (Lewis being the 'producer' and Jack a leading
member of the cast), taking discussion groups, chairing quizzes,
leading the daily sing-song, and acting on the committee.

They both saw themselves as the natural, although non-elected,
representatives of the participants. They asserted that this capacity
was theirs by virtue of their high level of involvement, and the fact
that they had no other interests in their lives but the Centre. This
was the basis for the frequent discords the couple had with
members of staff in which the main argument put forward by them
was that as members of staff focused their lives outside the Centre,

they had no real understanding of the place of the Centre in the lives of the participant and, therefore, were not in a position to take decisions on the running of the establishment.

Other participants who took the same view gathered around the two and as they both took a special interest in 'converting' new-comers into participants, their group was constantly enhanced (see 'Initiation'). Rifts with other participants provoked by their domi-nating manner and self-opinionated way of expression, and the countless activities in which they were involved, gave them an unpalatable reputation for power seeking.

In this respect Lewis and Jack's group was different from Alan's. Although sharing the same convictions about the impor-tance of the Centre in their lives, Alan and his friends refrained from any active attempt to change the running of the Centre. On several occasions they voiced criticisms, for instance on extending Centre activities, and the merger with the Jewish Blind Society centre, but they never tried to take Lewis and Jack's line, challenging and defying staff and contriving to take over partici-pants.

This difference in behaviour was partly due to the predominance of a fatalistic attitude amongst members of Alan's group. They rejected any possibility of premeditated change and argued that relations between events were entirely beyond the participants' control. This outlook was expressed in the daily gatherings of the group, Alan and his friends sitting cosily together in the buffer zone between the men and the women in the upper hall, chatting and occasionally singing. Any participant who felt like it could join the daily meetings and participate in the conversation and atmosphere without any difficulty. On the other hand, no attempts were made to gain new recruits, and the turnover was fairly high, although the hard core of Alan and three of his friends remained unchanged.

Discontent with staff or participants was rarely expressed. The only orthodoxy was the code of values of the care system. That was used as a major criterion for judging participants, evaluating activities and assessing relationships with staff and other participants.

Without exception, the stalwarts of the group were people who had disengaged themselves completely from pre-Centre forms of life. Most of them were living on their own in bedsitters or small flats, quite a number of them had strongly renounced their families, and all of them considered the possibility of taking up a new job and re-integrating into the outside world as inconceivable. This particular characteristic made possible the only significant breach in the strict separation between men and women in the Centre.

The other part of the upper hall was occupied by women engaging in craftwork and gossip. Most of them share the main characteristics of the women participants described previously, but a few were outstandingly different as their background suggested a long period of social isolation and disengagement. This created a recognized common ground with Alan's group and, indeed, the similarities in their situations became the basis for contact between the two.

It started when one of the women was heard bitterly complaining about her loneliness and emotional distress. Alan who was within earshot approached and asked her out to his local 'pub', a proposal which was gladly accepted. That incident marked the initiation of a more permanent friendship between the two, which made the woman an integral part of the group. Thenceforth other women gradually followed and within approximately a month Alan's group changed into a mixed daily gathering of men and women. Most of the women did not seem to be tempted by the opportunity to bridge the distance with the men by joining the group. They carried on working in the other part of the upper hall paying no apparent attention to the songs, jokes, gossip and small talk amongst the group.

A complete lack of mingling marked the relationship between Alan's group and the fourth identified group of participants. This consisted of Joel (see 'The ultimate reality'), Sam (see 'Alternative realities'), Joseph (see 'The idea of care') and a few others. All of them regarded their stay in the Centre strictly as an ephemeral phase in their lives – a transitory stage between the pre-Centre situation and a more desirable state. They visualized this future in different terms. Joel and others pictured their future in materialistic terms, of change in environment and means, while Joseph and Sam were concerned more with the spiritual level of their existence. Nevertheless, they all shared the same basic attitude that the Centre was a necessary evil. Consequently they refused to take part in activities, and looked down on other participants and rarely entered into conversation with them. This seemingly aloof and conceited behaviour provoked other participants, who pointed to the discrepancy between their condescending attitude and the reality, which put them in the same need of charity as the rest. The members of the group formed their own closed system of care which in fact (see 'The idea of care') resembled significantly patterns of exchange in the outside world. Nevertheless, despite their basic rejection of the Centre as a permanent solution, they all applauded the principles of the care system and hence did not face an attitude of ostracism and avoidance similar to that expressed towards participants like Rebecca (see 'Guarding the system'), who actively defied the system.

The rejection of the Centre as a viable alternative reality was most emphatically expressed by Joel, who was responsible for the emergence of the group with its distinctive membership, location and behaviour. Having been a relatively well-to-do business man, married to a local councillor and thus involved in community life, Joel was forced to join the Centre following a contest in a court case over the execution of his wife's will. After the Court decision he was planning to leave the area and find permanent accommodation in a seaside hotel for the elderly, and this he made known to participants as well as to staff. His disparaging remarks on the Centre ('A place of humiliation', 'hell', etc.) were attributed by participants to his bereavement and, therefore, did not arouse a reaction of avoidance and disengagement on their part. For his part, Joel did everything in his power to display his contempt for and detachment from the Centre people. Surrounded by books, 'serious' newspapers and publications, and producing letters and photographs associating him with certain dignitaries, such as the Chief Rabbi, members of parliament and even the royal family, Joel confined himself to an armchair, continuously passing snide remarks on the rest of the participants.

Gradually he was left to his incessant moaning and groaning. At that stage Joel established his first contacts with Joseph and Sam who, sharing his low regard for other participants, resigned themselves to voluntary seclusion around Joel's corner. In no time they found common ground, and a strong link was formed between them. They lunched together, supported each other in confronting other participants as well as staff, and established their exclusive system of mutual help.

Despite this overt disengagement a few attempts were made by Lewis and Jack to 'convert' them to their idea of participation. This seemed to meet with some success when individuals in the group were in a pessimistic mood about the fulfilments of their aspirations, but as soon as the chances of their plans materializing improved, they once again disassociated themselves from the others.

Most of the participants could not be identified with any of these groups. The majority hovered between meetings and gatherings, not committing themselves to any regular form of encounter and usually simply being welcomed by the permanent members of the groups, who did not look upon them as potential recruits but rather as recipients of attention and care.

Undoubtedly the balance between out-Centre orientation and a Centre-focused outlook was considerably affected by the life-histories of participants. Nevertheless, it should be noted that the convictions ingrained in the care system, the personal opportunities offered by the social reconstruction of time, and the mechanics of inculcating and controlling these notions, presented a real pressure on participants. Only a few held on to their former views and remained impervious to the Centre social reality.

The care system, although embracing the great majority of participants, varies in intensity and draws differential commitment from different individuals and groups. The dominance of the new conception of time varies with it. The less weight given to external commitments, the greater the impact of the care system and the new conception of the relation between events is. Conversely, the greater the external commitments, the smaller the impact of care relations, and the greater the likelihood of a return to the old, incongruous conceptions of time. Hence the differentiation of participants contributes to making the Centre a dynamic, ever-changing social reality.

Guarding the system

The coherence and legitimacy of the care system and its distilled time perspectives are vulnerable to three factors: (a) penetration into the Centre of contradictory concepts, which represent a direct cognitive threat to Centre values; (b) disagreements and discord between groups and individuals which might endanger the very basis of its existence; and (c) renegade individuals who, by

displaying behaviour and attitudes incompatible with the acceptable code of participation, introduce uncertainty and confusion
into the system. The way each potential threat is encountered and
treated will be the subject of this section.

An integral component of the atmosphere in the Centre is joke-
making and joking. There is some consistency as to what is good
for 'a laugh'; certain elements are recurrently used while others are
ignored. One can identify these elements primarily as those representing some intrusion of undesirable reminders of pre-Centre
situations, and out-Centre reality, or incongruities and ambiguities,
into the care system.

The reappearance of elements of the public, social definition of
old age, which were eliminated in the Centre, usually provoke a
joking reaction. A call to attend 'keep fit' classes was received with
a roar of laughter and ironic remarks. 'If I am fit enough!' 'You
will have to carry me there!' Able-bodied participants who
obtrusively displayed their fitness were frequently mocked, while
handicapped participants who could not take part in certain daily
Centre activities used irony to describe their plight. Thus in
response to the announcement of a dance, a crippled participant
pointed to his crutch and legs and said: 'And I am going to be the
prima ballerina.' He was told by a participant in a wheelchair, 'You
look as if you have just come from a dancing lesson.' Dances were
an acceptable arena for joking and mockery. Participants deliberately exaggerated their clumsiness and inability to keep time with
the music, displaying their walking aids and advertising their
awkwardness.

The awareness of disablement as one of the major constituents of
the social definition of old people pervaded most of the jokes in the
Centre's magazine, all of them paraphrases of well-known jokes,
such as the following dialogue, which takes place at a restaurant:

Guest (to an elderly waiter): 'Have you got matza balls?'
Waiter: 'This is the way I walk.'

Other 'humorous' pieces are meant to relate to the immediate
environment of participants, and include alongside references to
physical disabilities, references to another important stereotype –
the imputation of senility and confusion to the old. One such story
taken from *News and Views* manifests this:

Two gentlemen from the convalescent home went for a walk.

After a few minutes the younger man named Harry asked to be excused. The elder man named Sam said 'I will wait for you on the seat nearby.' After waiting ten minutes Sam went into the convenience and shouted out 'Are you alright Harry?' Harry replied 'Yes, why?' Sam said 'I have waited so long I thought you had fallen down the hole.' After a lengthy silence Harry said 'Don't be silly. How can I fall down the hole? I am too big.'

Behaviour associated with disorientation and confusion was a common cause of mirth, and the very mention of 'madness' and particularly 'senility' provoked laughter. It should be noted, however, that such references were never made by the participants themselves, but occurred when members of staff, or occasionally outsiders, accidently let them slip. The response could be interpreted in terms of Douglas's (1968) analysis of the joke as a means of social control.

Other scourges of old age such as loneliness were not treated as a subject for joking. The confidence expressed by participants in the power of the Centre environment to alleviate this problem and to integrate its 'treatment' into the care system presented no contradiction or incongruity.

Perhaps the major source for laughter in the Centre was the subject of sex amongst the elderly. Being well aware of society's denial of the possibility of sexual relationships in later years, the participants used to elaborate on the gap between the socially conceived impotence of old people and the desirable situation. Self-mockery and deliberate gross devaluation of present abilities relative to past sexual experience were common.

Joking, sardonic remarks such as 'I have got only one problem with sex: I do not get it' or 'I look worried today because I've forgotten to take my pill' are frequently exchanged alongside with numerous jokes, puns, limericks and rhymes all based on that perceived discrepancy. One noteworthy example is a local adaptation of a well-known anecdote, published in the participants' magazine:

A friend of mine living near Finsbury Park would see through her window an elderly man and woman who looked well over eighty, going into the park each day, always holding arms lovingly. One day she met them just as they were entering the park and stopped them saying 'I watch you every day from my window and I always think it wonderful to see how lovingly you hold arms still at your age.' The old lady answered: 'Don't be silly, we hold on to each other in case we fall.'

The realization that elderly people are excluded from the mainstream of life in society expresses itself by laughing at the possibility of attempting to restore contacts. Participants who talked about getting a job and resuming their working life were laughed at, as were participants who mentioned re-marriage, the revitalization of family relationships, or reintegration into the community. A cynical presentation of such attitudes also appeared in *News and Views*: 'What is an optimist? A man of seventy who marries a girl of nineteen and looks out for a new house near a shul' (slang for 'synagogue'). When the deputy supervisor asked participants to put their names down for personal New Year greeting cards (devised and executed by Jonathan, who was the builder and operator of the Centre's printing machine), he was greeted with a roar of laughter. There was a scanty response, as to almost any other initiative associated with the Jewish community. Any mention of the affluent Jewish community in north-west London aroused snide remarks and jokes, and so did any talk of prominent figures in the Jewish establishment.

Three areas were exempted from this overall devaluation of Jewish institutions. The first was the nostalgic view of East End life (see 'Revising the past'), the second was Israel (see 'Alternative realities'), and the third was the Nazi holocaust and its victims, some of whom attended the Centre.

On the other hand, any incongruity with Centre reality was the subject of mockery. A woman who claimed in a speech during the public speaking competition that a relation of hers had made his money on his own initiative, through his ingenuity, thus openly questioning the fatalistic point of view held by participants, was laughed at and, needless to say, eliminated from the contest. A participant who said that he had been at a tombstone laying ceremony for one of his friends was told that 'children set up a stone only to prevent their dead parents from getting up again'. Participants who showed respect for religious institutions were often laughed at, and soon learnt to keep their beliefs to themselves.

Inadvertent, slight abuses of the care-system principles were also treated as jokes. This refers mostly to people who comply with the overall concept of care, but for one reason or another unwillingly or unwittingly deviate from one of its principles. This mainly applies to married couples who present a contradiction to the element of non-personal exchange (see 'Patterns of care'). When the identity of a couple obtrudes, the usual response is an apologetic self-mocking one. Thus a woman who was asked what she would do in the event of her husband being kidnapped replied, 'I would pay them to keep him.' A couple who met at the Centre and decided to get married became the subject of countless jokes. Participants speculated about the couple's sexual relationship and expressed their belief that they both suffered from some emotional instability. Such comments were usually accompanied by vivid 'examples' to corroborate the assumption that the only reason for the marriage was sheer stupidity. The couple, well aware of this attitude, spent extra efforts to reinforce their status as care renderers.

The prominence of care can pose a problem of self-evaluation for participants who are unable to help. The care system caters for such cases, attenuating feelings of guilt and creating opportunities for demonstrating help despite physical handicaps (see 'Patterns of care'), but participants are still faced with the need to explain to themselves and to others their limitations as helpers. This was often done by ironic self-reproach. 'You see, they couldn't work without my help, could they? It's good to know I am around.'

One could not, however, make light of the care system itself. Thus a member of the concert party entertainment group who proclaimed that the rehearsals and the mistakes made by the performers should not be taken seriously as 'It is only for fun', was angrily expelled from the cast.

Joking is not always sufficient to blur discords and contradictions. Interaction between participants often involved confrontations which could have engendered long-standing disputes. However, this happened rarely. The general pattern was of a short outburst, which subsided with no noticeable long term impact on the relationship. In fact this form of encounter was so common in the Centre that participants accepted it as a normal part of the interaction between them, though more than once they sought the advice of staff when, in the heat of the moment, violent reactions were provoked.

Most of the outbursts in the Centre were the result of clashes over power. As the striving for power and authority was structurally a disruptive element to the care system, attempts to exercise power immediately provoked an outburst. Thus when the organizer of the concert party tried to limit the number of members of cast, a woman participant, who decided that she had the right to appear in the show, started shouting and screaming. The participants persuaded the organizer to give in and allow the woman to join the cast. In fact, by conceding to this demand the organizer avoided the struggle over influence and allowed the situation to revert to its care-setting, characterized by the lack of leadership.

Membership of the committee always provoked accusations and counter-accusations about attempts to establish leadership. At times, especially at general meetings, this led to demands to remove certain members because of their excessively authoritative manner in performing their tasks. They were accused of 'bullying' participants, 'dictating' and 'being governors'. Invariably such outbursts lasted no more than a few minutes and ended in reconciliation based on a reiterated pledge that committee membership does not entail a position of authority, a pledge usually accepted with the words, 'I have got nothing against you.'

Inside the committee, discords followed the same pattern. After recriminations, someone would either leave the room in a raging temper or throw his papers on the floor and swear not to participate in the committee any longer. A third party, usually the supervisor, Jonathan or other peace-makers, would get the contenders together, praise them both for their goodwill and devotion to the Centre, and ask them to forget all about the row. This would normally be sufficient to restore the relationship, until the next outburst.

Much effort and consideration were invested by participants in the avoidance of disputes. This was done either by shifting a possible focus for conflict from participants to staff, or by isolating it in another way from the multiplexity of relationships between participants. The first solution was employed when the source of discord was complaints concerning the running of the Centre, the activities, transport and lunch arrangements, etc. In such cases participants were instantly referred to members of staff whilst receiving full backing from the referee – usually a member of the committee. Assertions such as 'It is none of our business' or 'We can't help the way they run the Centre' were commonly made in such situations.

Discontents were unavoidable where the management of the 'benevolent fund', or other functions under the participants' own initiative, were concerned. Two complementary strategies were employed to tackle such occurrences. The first was to insist that whatever happened the disagreement should not affect the relationship between the parties involved. If this strategy failed and a participant was determined to carry on fighting, the other people involved would usually avoid him or ignore his presence.

In most instances discord was contained. Crises, although appearing to be the emotional climax to a tense situation, arose consistently in response to various temporary needs in the Centre. Thus shouting people down to enable a discussion or a talk to continue, expressing minority opinions, reacting to personal offences, contradicting 'outrageous' assertions (such as 'You are too young to attend the Centre' or other discriminating remarks), were all provoked by a potential incongruity in the care system, in the form of inequality, competition over resources, and factious tendencies among participants.

Relationships with staff were also liable to erupt into outbursts, and scenes in which participants complained at the tops of their voices about various aspects of the Centre management were quite common. The causes for such incidents covered a wide spectrum of subjects ranging from the quality of food, sitting arrangements, subjects for discussion groups and social work, to general confusion relating to policies and trends in the overall running of the establishment. Disagreements over areas of authority, such as the control of volunteers, arrangements for outings, layout of activities, etc., also quite commonly resulted in brief public rows.

Most of the participants were well aware of this mode of behaviour and when asked to explain its prevalence in the Centre interpreted it as a form of 'emotional reaction', 'nerves', or even 'a disease'. They all accepted that it would be pointless and unwise to try and restrain people from expressing themselves in such a fashion, as one cannot suppress and control one's emotions. In this way, outbursts became an acceptable target for help and concern, and thus an integral part of the care system, rather than a disruptive element.

The acceptance of the brief row but not the long term dispute has far-reaching implications for the organization of events in the Centre, and so for the constitution of time. As disputes, unlike outbursts, involve long term relationships, calculated actions and anticipation, they would imply a past-future conception of time. By resorting to outbursts this possible incongruity in the time-perspective of the Centre is forestalled.

When participants question the fundamentals of the Centre reality by persisting in the pursuit of certain forms of dissident behaviour and ideas, they run the risk of being avoided by the rest of the participants. Reasons for excluding people from full participation are varied and include constant, deliberate disruption of craft work; coming to the Centre only for lunches; giving an impression of being wealthy and not in need; and the expression of anti-Israeli opinions. A person was ostracized only after a long period of consistent, challenging behaviour. Being ostracized was usually merely a stage in a process of being driven out from the Centre.

Rebecca was known to be an irritable, cantankerous participant, but this did not single her out from other participants who were also nervous and defiant. What made her a target for contempt and avoidance was a combination of the way she expressed her conception of her place in the Centre, and her opinion of the rest of the participants. Lunch time was the usual occasion for Rebecca to protest about the food, the company of her co-diners, the state of cleanliness of the cutlery, the service, and almost anything else conceivable. Her judgments were considered to be outrageous. She constantly made caustic remarks about the fate of the Jews during the Nazi holocaust, proclaiming that they had deserved extermination, and that the people in the Centre had, unfortunately, had a lucky escape. She was nicknamed 'Mrs Hitler' by the participants. Her condescending, genteel mannerisms increased the hostility towards her, and her frequent mention of her family, her past wealth, and her cultured upbringing, contrasted to what she regarded as the 'bad stock' of the participants, deepened the general distaste.

The reaction of the participants suggested the social mechanism behind witchcraft accusations. Rebecca was held responsible for the abolition of the special gastric diet, for keeping would-be participants away from the Centre, and for spreading malicious gossip about the participants outside the Centre. Participants told of unpleasant encounters with her whilst queuing up for buses, and on the buses. They all stressed that her objectionable manners were renowned in all quarters of the local community, and damaged the Centre's reputation. In effect, the impression was that participants set Rebecca apart as an object for hatred, representing all despised out-Centre worldly attributes. It was as if she made manifest the clear-out boundaries between a 'participant' and the outside, time-bound old person.

Her ostracism was total. She was never offered a seat even when it was obvious that she could not stand – an act which was contradictory in nature to the idea of care, but fully congruent with the rigidity of the care system and its consistency. Her attempts to initiate occasional conversations with participants were completely ignored and her persistent effort to provoke some reaction by shouting, complaining and moaning were to no avail. She was approached several times by members of staff who asked her to try and get on with the participants, and as the tension grew a few participants expressed their desire to remove her forcibly from the Centre. Rebecca was then requested to leave the place for good, which she did.

Whereas Rebecca by her behaviour rejected the idea of participation and the care system, Martin seemed to have tried to do just the opposite and yet he was also ostracized. Martin was established in the area as a professional pauper or *schnorrer*. He was known to go around knocking on doors begging for money and old clothes. When he initially attended the Centre it was purely for the meals and the tea. He showed no interest whatsoever in other participants or in their activities. Nevertheless, he gradually showed signs of attempting to involve himself. He told jokes, joined the daily 'sing-along' and gave his unsought advice on dealing with the authorities and the social services – both matters on which he was an indisputable expert. Trouble arose when Martin started 'to deliberately interrupt' activities and conversations by proclaiming his opinions, challenging participants to include him, and trying to instigate rows and hostility between them. Although ignored, Martin was not taken aback by his exclusion. The critical turning point came when one of the participants accused Martin outright of being a pauper, living on charity and, therefore, disgracing the Centre by his presence. Other participants supported him and demanded Martin's removal from the Centre. Some of them went so far as to threaten the use of violence if he did not choose to go of his own accord. Like Rebecca, Martin disappeared from the Centre scene.

Both Rebecca and Martin represented breaches of the Centre's boundaries with the outside world and, therefore, were not eligible for inclusion in the care system. Rebecca sinned by judging the participants in terms of a system of statuses, hierarchies and time which they rejected, Martin by his stigmata of shame and indignity which participants endeavoured to obliterate. Thus they both breached the boundary between participants and the outside world, representing an intrinsic incongruity which could not be tolerated.

In most instances people passed through the process of becoming participants without upsetting the intricate relationship between the Centre and the outside world. None the less, this relationship constituted the major axis around which initiation into the participants' community, as well as the social differentiation between them, revolved. This perceived contrast between the reality outside and the Centre life should be examined in the light of the temporal properties it contains.

The transition from a past-future orientated society to a present-bound community is a well-regulated process, and so is the daily interaction and grouping among participants. A participant faces a clear-cut choice between identifying himself – in word and action – with the principles of the social reality in the Centre or else with those of the world outside. No compromise is acceptable, and one is not allowed to make the most of both worlds. A participant is required to demonstrate publicly and decisively his allegiance and commitment to the Centre. In this respect the experience of participation is total and indivisible, and the submergence of the individual into a new time universe makes a complete, coherent change in his existence.

Conclusions: The Centre time universe – a theoretical perspective

Anthropological theorizing about time perspective and time reckoning schemes is still in the formative stage. The cross-cultural study has not yet even been given a name nor have schools of thought about the subject emerged within the discipline (Maxwell, 1972, pp. 47-8).

The temporal properties embedded in the participants' social world pose a variety of sociological questions, which demand special attention; particularly since I wish to suggest that the examination of the temporal dimension in people's lives will always provide us with important clues to their worldview and behavioural patterns.

1

The sharp contrast between the Centre and the outside indicates that the participants' community acts as a viable alternative reality both to previous experience and to present, external contingencies. The social world of the Centre offers to the neophyte participant a total solution to his existential problems. The time-perspective ingrained in this counter-world is also comprehensive, in the sense that all its ingredients are congruent with one another, and represent a coherent system of reordering one's time universe.

Roth (1963, p. 114) suggests that 'If one wishes to apply a time-table analysis to a whole of a person's life, he must realise that each person operates on a number of timetables simultaneously', but it is plausible that the apparently divergent timetables stem from a single, fairly consistent worldview. However, the pre-Centre situation as described in the first chapter confronted the aged with a discrepant time universe deriving from two incongruent realities – the world of the non-aged versus the actual state of the aged. For this the Centre substituted an experience of time which was as total and as coherent as the social system of which it was a part.

A viable analytical starting point is simply to spell out the composition of the Centre time universe, bearing in mind the normally expected patterns of ordering time. There is an almost taken-for-granted premise that any time-perspective should consist of three consecutive elements – past, present and future.

> Future, present and past exist with respect of one another in the same manner as the terms of an infinite series (Dunne, 1939, 1938).

> If the series is broken by removing a term or terms so that the remaining term or terms stand alone, they lose their meaning. If the present is removed or if the future and past are simultaneously eliminated a state of unbeing should result (Aaronson, 1972, p. 408).

The socially eliminated past and future of the Centre people certainly did not create a 'state of unbeing'. On the contrary, one might say that the attempt to eliminate past and future permits a renewal of the participants' social 'being'.

The emphasis on the present and neglect of past and future is by no means new in the study of human behaviour. Doob (1971, p. 409) contemplates the possibility of a present-bound society where 'only absorption in the moment counts; the past cannot really be recaptured; the future cannot be controlled'. Lévi-Strauss (1967, pp. 233-4) suggests:

> that the distinction between people without history, and others could with advantages be replaced with a distinction between what for convenience I called 'cold' and 'hot' societies, the former seeking by the institutions they give themselves, to annul the possible effects of historical factors on their equilibrium and continuity in a quasi-automatic fashion, the latter resolutely internalizing the historical process and making it the moving power of their development.

Bohannan (1953) found among the Tiv of Nigeria that the concept of casuality is non-existent, and that time is marked by the juxta-position of two events. Beidelman (1963) describes two distinct temporal sequences among the Kaguru of East Africa, the first a very detailed and specified one referring to a period of less than a

day, the second, referring only to major events of the past, lacking
continuity and intervals. This is a society living by the cycle of
nature almost regardless of past and future events. Similar reports
have come from students of some modern western groups. Seeley *et
al.*, (1956, p. 5) discovered that the people of Crestwood Heights
'live almost entirely in the present but for the near future, with the
past largely obliterated'. The attitudes towards time of a hippie
community reveals a conception of time rooted in a nihilistic worldview. 'Why plan if all plans can disintegrate into a nuclear dust?'
(Davis, 1967, p. 15). A conception of the world which 'prompts a
radical shift in time perspective – from what will be to what is.
From future promise to present fulfilment ...' (ibid.). Comparable
time perspectives could be found in other so-called deviant groups
such as alcoholics (Button, 1956) and drug users (Cheek and
Laucius, 1972). Cheek and Laucius even suggest that this approach
to life distinguishes the outlook of a whole new generation (ibid.,
p. 344).

2

I treated the arrest of time in the Centre, and the formation of a
present-oriented society as a reaction to a temporal incongruity
rather than as a chance development. Hence, time was treated as an
existential problem, a problem as deserving of sociological analysis
as status inconsistency, role conflict or cultural ambiguity. This
runs counter to the traditional conception of time as a mere by-
product of social life. I agree with Doob (1971, p. 406) that
'Temporal orientation, temporal information and temporal
standards can play a critical role in behaviour.'

   This role is perhaps most evident in social situations and
sequences of events where some disorder takes place. One possibility is the emergence of a discontinuity in a consecutive series of
events, or a breach in the relationship between past, present and
future. Another possibility is the emergence of an incongruity or
inconsistency in the social norms patterning one's time-perspective
at a given point in one's life.

   Much of the relevant psychological and socio-anthropological
literature is concerned primarily with problems in the life cycle (for
example: Erikson, 1959; Jung, 1971; Kuhlen, 1964; Peck, 1956). A
recapitulation of the main theme of this work is provided by Doob:

Time is irreversible, as is so often sadistically indicated. You will never be young again, yes and you know that your body will age, and that other persons and circumstances will change. If you wish to summarize all this with the concept of time, well and good, but to some extent you are oversimplifying and are personifying the concept. Many other occasions therefore, on which time must be noted, are the ones which cannot be reversed and to that extent frustration and temporal judgment of despair are invoked. In addition the limiting case of death faces us all and hence noting our age – after, let us say, the bloom begins to fade – is bound to be frustrating to some extent, from which circumstance generalization to many other aspects of time may well occur (Doob, 1971, p. 92).

The irreversibility of time has been presented as the crux of a major existential problem faced, particularly, by the aged. This line of research stresses the inability of the old to change their environment or to influence their own fate, yet the Centre people not only did construct a new social reality, but by doing so also offered a solution to the problem of irreversibility.

The possibility of arresting time has captured the imagination of many writers, and is expressed in various literary and intellectual forms. Nevertheless, research into its possible implementation in reality is scanty. Doob (1971, p. 239) entertains the idea, suggesting that:

> The old ... wish to delay the future, to hold back time; they know that they have lived a long while, they may feel that they have not accomplished as much as they have once wished and they are compelled to realize that increasingly few opportunities remain before they die.

Adaptation mechanisms based on alteration in time perspective were described by Davis (1967) and Horton (1967) in the context of young adults' behaviour – the former dealing with hippies and the latter with the street culture of blacks. In both instances the insignificance of the past and vague prospects for the future led to an emphasis on the present, and something similar may be discerned in the situation of the participants in the day centre. None the less, one is bound to ask whether this line of interpretation – i.e. comparing the relevance of the three components of time to one another – is a satisfactory way of approaching the whole subject of alteration in time perspective.

Some of the most important sources of the participants' conceptions of time derived not from the relationship between past, present and future, but from the actual, existential situation they experienced. In other words, the incongruities and ambiguities of the limbo state were predominant factors in constituting the Centre's time universe. Thus, in order to gain a better understanding of the nature of the 'solution' developed in the Centre to the problem of time, a situational analysis is necessary. The diachronic perspective must be complemented by a synchronic, even though the subject under discussion is seemingly by definition 'diachronic'.

Traces of such an approach may be detected in a few studies, perhaps most constructively in the suggestion of Roth (1963) and his followers that

> people will not accept uncertainty, they will make an effort to structure it, no matter how poor the materials they have to work with and no matter how much the experts try to discourage them. One way to structure uncertainty is to structure the time period through which uncertain events occur (ibid., p. 93).

The study on the Centre people showed that rather than just facing uncertainty, the participants confronted a breach in their time universe. Such breaches in the social position of the aged were noted by Neugarten (1968); Riley (1971); and Foner (1975), who wrote:

> social aging (age mobility) need not be underestimated. For each increment in years of life there is no necessary increment in social rewards. Much depends on the special structure of age-stratification in any given society .... The greatest rewards accrue to those strata which are chronologically in the middle. This means that age mobility as a social phenomenon is curvilinear in modern society. People tend to be upwardly mobile in many respects (that is move to positions with increasingly social rewards) well through the middle years but thereafter they tend to become downwardly mobile, as social rewards are widely withdrawn or reduced. Such loss of rewards, typically involuntary, may engender in the old the same sense of despair found

among other deprived groups who see no chance of improving their lot (ibid., p.157).

I would like to suggest that such incongruity between age and social position should not be viewed only in terms of rewards and stratification, but also as a cognitive ambiguity created by the incompatibility between personal experience and social conceptions. The Centre people did not enjoy a life cycle of achievements and increasing social approval. Nevertheless, their experience of the incongruous temporal dimension in their later life was severe.

3

What are, in Roth's terms, 'the materials' of the new reality constructed in the Centre? What is the nature of the relationship between those materials?

Evidently the substance we are dealing with is human interaction, but such interaction must be analysed according to the underlying themes uniting its independent components into a meaningful reality. The major theme in this case is the unique conception of time underpinning the interpersonal relationships in the Centre. Time, therefore, becomes the cardinal constituent of the participants' behaviour. Thus time is viewed in this context not as a mere reflection of a certain social reality nor even as just another problem in people's lives. I suggest that time must be viewed as a viable, manipulable resource open to infinite possibilities of handling and management through people's attitudes and behaviour.

Time was perceived as a resource in a number of studies relating to various social environments. Thus Cohen and Taylor (1972) ascribe to it the attributes of an important resource in prison life. Smith (1961, p.85) suggests that time 'occupies a people's thought to such an extent that the measurements of time may become a preoccupation. To such a society time is a commodity to be spent, lost, invested, saved, wasted, drowned away or employed to "best advantage".' Calkins (1970, p.487) suggests 'Time is planned, allotted, clipped, saved and spent in order that priorities are met.' However, people in the Centre do not express this manipulation of time in temporal terminology. The constitution of their conception is inherent in their social world and one has to elicit it and to translate it into conventional conceptual frameworks of time analysis.

The manipulation of time in the Centre is implemented neither by altering the codes of a time reckoning system, nor by artificial experimental restructuring of the temporal perception of one's mind and personality (for example, by hypnosis – Aaronson, 1972 – or by means of administering certain drugs – Cheek and Laucius, 1972). Nor is it done by resorting to the world of dreams, the arts or the supernatural (Doob, 1971, pp.370 – 412). The participants manipulated time by using the social system they created, a social system which did not include an explicit method for reckoning, measuring and conceptualizing, but nevertheless contained a major alteration of their temporal orientation.

This last point raises the most crucial issue of the relationship between time and society. The terms of the controversy were summarized by Maxwell (1972. p.50) as follows:

> there are two processes in handling time. One ... is that of the behavioural expression of the time perspective in its ordinary sense of selective emphasis on past, present or future events. The other ... is that of ordering time or measuring it in units.

In other words the issue in question is whether time is a behavioural factor or merely an abstraction of a system of ordering events and dividing socio-ecological units. Obviously, the two perspectives do not necessarily stand in sharp contrast to each other and there is a large area of overlap. Nevertheless, the discussion in the anthropological literature diverges into two distinct lines of approaching time. The first is the massive ethnography on time reckoning as a cultural reflection of either ecological conditions (Malinowski, 1927; Nilsson, 1920) or a social system (Evans-Pritchard, 1939, 1940; Sorokin and Merton, 1937) or both (Maltz, 1968). The other line is founded on the premise that the time perspective is basic in any social system and its exploration vital to the understanding of the basic characteristics of that culture (for examples, Kluckhohn, 1953; Kluckhohn and Strodtbeck, 1961; Hall, 1959, 1966).

As will be obvious from this study, I view time not only as an essential determinant of the participants' social world, but as also the foundation on which this world was built. Thus, any attempt to overlook the importance of the temporal dimension or to underestimate it will result in a miscomprehension of the nature of that social reality.

Finally, Leach (1966, p.125) and Barnes (1971) have defined two recurrent elements in conceptions of time. One involves the notion of irreversibility, of directional change, the other involves the notion of repetition, of cycles of events. The transformation of the constitution of time in the Centre depends upon a stress on the repetitive element. The irreversible aspect of time is cognitively obliterated. However, unusually perhaps, this repetitive pattern of events is not thought of as being cyclical. The separate units of time do not follow in any sequence, but rather constitute independent units. The metaphor of the pendulum (rather than the arrow or the cycle) is an apt representation of Centre time.

The movement from the anomic and incongruous time perspective which characterizes the limbo state to the coherent time universe of the Centre involves far more than just an alteration in the constitution of events. A fundamental change in references, values and outlook underlie the new conception.

The Centre presents a sharp contrast to the values and the ways of the outside world, and in content and structure it represents an alternative, viable social reality. The repetitive nature of events, coupled with the more verbally explicit revision of the past and the obliteration of the future, create a new constitution of time in which change is arrested and progress and planning are eliminated; and yet people find themselves doing meaningful, purposeful things within a well-defined, structured social arena. The change-proof environment is not stagnant, nor is it aimless and anomic. Without the support of a system of beliefs in the supernatural, and with no references to external forces, the people of the Centre have created a new way of responding to a whole gamut of existential incongruities and ambiguities which are commonly considered unavoidable and inexorable.

As a social phenomenon rather than a sociological issue, the world of the participants challenges a number of widespread social images of the aged. It brings into question the alleged inflexibility of old people, their supposed inability to change their environment and existential conditions, and the belief that segregation and lack of involvement with the non-aged are detrimental to the satis-faction and contentment people experience in their later years. The possible implication of these findings (granted that each case is examined on its own particular merits) for social policy, the organization of welfare services and community work may be far reaching, and I leave them to the reader's consideration.

Methodological notes

Studying a day centre, it was obviously necessary to encompass as far as possible the life of participants in the outside world. I was tempted to follow the ramification of outside relationships, such as family networks, relationships within the community, class identifications, religious affiliations, relations with neighbours, friends etc. In principle all might be relevant to the main line of the argument, and, indeed, most were taken into account. The difficulty was rather where to stop, what to exclude. In the end the fieldwork strategy was shaped largely by the exigencies of the situation.

My initial attempt to act the role of an uncommitted observer soon proved to be impractical. This was a consequence of the very nature of the Centre, and the distinct boundary between 'in' and 'out', 'participants' and 'others'. You either conformed to the rules of the care system etc. governing the relationship there – in that event full commitment and active involvement were required – or your presence would have been obliterated. The choice of a middle-of-the-road position did not exist.

This division between 'in' and 'out' overrode other preconceived distinctions. Thus, leaning on past experience and relevant ethnography, I tried not to identify myself with the staff, in the hope that such an attitude would promote my image as a disinterested party in the Centre. This just did not work, for the key to recognition and acceptance by participants was rather an evident approval of and commitment to the Centre reality. Only when I understood this principle and acted accordingly was I accepted as a friend and confidant, deserving to be treated on equal terms with the rest of the participants.

Objectivity, while I strained for it, had to some extent to be surrendered, for anything less than full assimilation in the Centre reality would have presented a serious impediment to the understanding of occurrences. Participants and staff alike made it clear by their behaviour that unless a committed attitude was expressed by me, the degree of co-operation and help rendered by them would not extend some formal reserved boundaries. As it happened, some of the most valuable pieces of information were gathered during events which one might describe as 'manufactured by the researcher'.

Personal involvement determined to a great extent the choice of attendance and observation. Sometimes apparently important activities had to be neglected, in favour of a simultaneously-held activity where participation was essential for the preservation of already established personal relationships. Consequently, an imbalance developed in sources of information from different sections of participants. Thus as I was 'initiated' and looked after mostly by the men upstairs, I could not devote a fair share of attention to the women upstairs and the disabled downstairs. My attempts to intensify relationships with these two categories were frowned on by my caretakers, who expected me to adopt their own attitudes towards the rest of the participants.

This feature of the research posed a serious difficulty during the last stage of fieldwork, when I combined participation in the Centre activities with regular sessions at the head office of the Jewish Welfare Board, browsing through the participants' records, and becoming acquainted with the organizational side. This split preoccupation, although explicitly appreciated by participants as a necessary step in the research, did not fit with the involvement in the Centre life, and strong disapproval was expressed. Participants questioned my full commitment and loyalty to their world. Inevitably, a process of disengagement started and a growing feeling of unpleasant suspicion and, perhaps, slight disappointment on the part of the participants took the place of the former welcoming, open and relaxed relationship.

The recognition of the time factor as the cornerstone for the analysis made me realize that a longitudinal study of the lives of the people in question is vital to the understanding of their present situation. None the less, as technically such a research was impossible, one can only speculate on the disadvantages and imperfections caused by its absence. Some partial remedies were, of course, available measures. The most important was the collection of autobiographies, supplemented by interviews with other contemporaries living in the area or known to be familiar with the world of East End Jewry. The participants' personal files, the annual reports of the Jewish Board of Guardians and some other written material contributed also to a clearer picture of the participants' life-histories.

My argument depended to some extent on an understanding of current attitudes to old people. Although a systematic cultural study of the position of the aged in society was beyond the scope of this study, I was able to elicit the impressions and conceptions of participants on this subject. This method of approach had the advantage of revealing the perceived social environment of the Centre people. This was complemented by observations of occasions in which the outside world penetrated the Centre, in the form of public talks, printed materials, activities organized by volunteers, and occasional visits by local dignitaries and other guests.

I would suggest in conclusion that while my personal involvement and the occasional need to appeal to inadequately established cultural assumptions might be felt to detract from the 'objectivity' of the study, my methods did permit a more complete insight into the Centre reality than would otherwise have been possible.

Notes

1 The limbo state

1   I confine the argument to the Centre population although there is little doubt in my mind that these characteristics apply to many other elderly populations in our society.

2   All data relating to the general Jewish population of Marlsden is based on *Jews in an Inner London Borough*, by Harvey A. Kosmin and Nigel Grizzard, published by the Statistical and Demographic Research Unit of the London Committee of the British Jews, March 1975.

3   Ibid., p.14.

4   This schematic description will be elaborated upon later.

5   'I am fine' by Vera G. Tyler, published in *A Newsletter for Disabled People Living in the London Borough of Marlsden*, vol.3, no.2, December 1973, p.3.

6   From 'On Retirement – A Lament' by A.I. Ling. Taken from *'News and Views'*, the day centre magazine, May 1973, p.18.

7   Printed in *News Letter*, December 1974 – a bulletin issued by the voluntary services section of the Jewish Welfare Board.

8   *Manifesto on the Place of the Retired and the Elderly in Modern Society*, published by 'Age Concern', England, 1975.

9   A term suggested by Gouldner (1973, p.296) to explain the imbalance in reciprocity between different sectors of society.

10   From *Day Care and Leisure Provisions for the Elderly*, an 'Age Concern' publication, 1974, p.6.

11   *Jewish Chronicle*, 4 April 1975, p.6.

12   'The Special Centre Song' by Florence Howson, taken from *A Newsletter for Disabled People Living in the London Borough of Marlsden*, vol.4, no.2, p.8, published by Marlsden Association for the Disabled.

13   For example, a homeless man who adheres to the belief that by his action he fulfils a divine mission in this world. They are isolated cases and have little impact on the other people in question.

14   In other instances, such as ethnic and racial groups, criminals and other social deviants, etc., it would seem that the social attitudes directed towards them also constitute and mould the actual conditions characterizing them. On the aged as a minority group, see for example Foner (1975).

15   For example, Kastenbaum (1963).

16   A further, more extended discussion on the temporal dimension in the relevant literature will be given in the concluding chapter.

2 The setting

1   'First Report on Jewish Welfare Board North-East London Day Centre', memo. by members of staff, August 1972, p.5.

2   In the course of the fieldwork several organizational and personnel changes
    took place, and they will be discussed later.
3   This arrangement changed a few times during the period of research. The
    reasons for this will be discussed later.
4   Taken from a report on the Centre written by members of staff, September
    1974, pp.2, 4, 5.
5   Ibid., p.6.
6   Before that time meals were provided free of charge. The nominal charge was
    introduced to 'retain the dignity of participants', and has since gone up three
    times to 25p.
7   Ibid., pp.3, 7, 8.
8   Ibid., p.8.
9   Ibid., pp.11, 12.
10 Ibid., p.9.
11 Background knowledge for this comparison derives from three main sources;
    (a) some acquaintance with the problems concerning the Board's old age
    homes: (b) relevant literature dealing with the characteristics of total institu-
    tions in general and old age homes in particular (Goffman, 1961; Sykes, 1966;
    Strauss *et al.*, 1963; Townsend, 1964; Bennett, 1963; Edgerton, 1963–4;
    Rosengren and Lefton, 1969); (c) research based on fieldwork carried out in an
    old age home in Israel (1972–3) under the supervision of Dr S. Deshen and
    Professor R. Shapira (MA thesis, Department of Sociology and Anthropology,
    Tel Aviv University).
12 Ibid., p.11
13 Ibid., p.9.
14 The first Centre supervisor is referred to henceforth as 'the supervisor' whereas
    his replacement will be called 'the new supervisor'.
15 I shall discuss further aspects of the management of the Centre in relation to
    the culture of the participants later.
16 Report on the Centre, September 1974, p.9.
17 Ibid., p.11.
18 Head office was situated in the West End of London until February 1975, and
    then it was transferred to the north-west. In both instances it was quite far
    from the Centre.

3   Reordering time

1   See relevant references to games at the Centre (ch.4, sec.3).
2   Jewish ritual lawfulness – especially in relation to food.
3   Official overseer appointed by the religious authorities to observe Kashrut
    restrictions.
4   The fact that the Lubavitz Rabbi emphasized the humane elements in the sect's
    ideology seemed to be overlooked by the audience. This could be accounted for
    by the intrinsic threat to the participants' conception of the uniqueness of the
    Centre's values as opposed to the negation of such values in the outside world,
    especially the idea of care and help. See ch.4.
5   Most of the Jewish Blind Society members were younger and, with the excep-
    tion of their eyesight, less handicapped than the Centre's participants.
6   'When I Must Leave You' by Hellen Steiner Rice, *Just for You (A Collection
    of Inspirational Verses)*, p.39. For further information see Case 1, 'Initiation'.

5   The limbo society

1   The belief in an after-life as such as a viable reality could be eliminated in view

of the attitude of obliteration and denial towards death prevailing in the Centre (see 'The ultimate reality').
2   This mixture of resemblances and dissimilarities might provide a line for a critique of Turner's (1967, 1969) discussion on the sociological nature of rites de passage.
3   'First report on J.W.B. North-East London Day Centre', pp.5-6.

References

AARONSON, B.S. (1972), 'Behaviour and the Future of Time', in H. Yaker, H. Osmond and F. Cheek (eds), *The Future of Time*, New York, Anchor, pp.405-36.

BARNES, J.A. (1971), 'Time Flies Like an Arrow', *Man* (NS) 6, pp.537-52.

BEIDELMAN, T.O. (1963), 'Kaguru Time Reckoning: An Aspect of the Cosmology of an East-African People', *Southwestern Journal of Anthropology*, 19, pp.9-20.

BENNETT, A.J. (1963), 'The Meaning of Institutional Life', *The Gerontologist*, 3, pp.117-25.

BERGER, P.L. and LUCKMANN, T. (1966), *The Social Construction of Reality*, Harmondsworth, Penguin.

BOHANNAN, P. (1953). 'Concepts of Time among the Tiv of Nigeria', *Southwestern Journal of Anthropology*, 9, pp.251-62.

BUTLER, R.N. (1964), 'The Life Review: An Interpretation of Reminiscences in the Aged' in R. Kastenbaum (ed.), *New Thoughts on Old Age*, New York, Springer, pp.265-90.

BUTTON, A.D. (1956), 'The Psychodynamics of Alcoholism: A Survey of 87 Cases', *Quarterly Journal of Studies in Alcohol*, 17, pp.296-305.

CALKINS, K. (1970), 'Time: Perspectives, Marking and Styles of Usage', *Social Problems*, 17, pp.487-501.

CHEEK, F.E. and LAUCIUS, J. (1972), 'The Time Worlds of Three Drug-Using Groups: Alcoholic Addicts, Heroin Addicts and Psychedelics' in H. Yaker, H. Osmond and F. Cheek (eds), *The Future of Time*, New York, Anchor, pp.230-45.

COHEN, P. (1972), *Subcultural Conflict and Working Class Community*, Working Paper in Cultural Studies, Centre for Contemporary Culture, University of Birmingham.

COHEN, S. and TAYLOR, L. (1972), *Psychological Survival*, Harmondsworth, Penguin.

CUMMING, E. and HENRY, W.E. (1961), *Growing Old: The Process of Disengagement*, New York, Basic Books.

DAVIS, F. (1967), 'Why All of Us may be Hippies Someday', *Trans-Action*, 5 (no.2.), pp.10-18.

DOOB, L. (1971), *Patterning of Time*, New Haven and London, Yale University Press.

DOUGLAS, M. (1968), 'The Social Control of Cognition: Some Factors in Joke Perception', *Man* (NS), 3, pp.361-77.

DUNNE, J.W. (1938), *This Serial Universe*, London, Macmillan.

DUNNE, J.W. (1939), *An Experiment with Time*, London, Faber & Faber.

EDGERTON, R.B. (1963-4), 'A Patient Elite: Ethnography in a Hospital for the Mentally Retarded', *American Journal of Mental Deficiency*, 68, pp.372-85.

ERIKSON, E. (1959), Identity and the Life Cycle, *Psychological Issues 1*, New York, International Press.

EVANS-PRITCHARD, E.E. (1939), 'Nuer Time Reckoning', *Africa*, 12, pp.189-216.

EVANS-PRITCHARD, E.E. (1940), *The Nuer*, Oxford University Press.

FONER, A. (1975), 'Age in Society – Structure and Change', *American Behavioral Scientist*, 19, pp.144-65.

GOFFMAN, E. (1961), 'On the Characteristics of Total Institutions', in his *Asylums*, New York, Anchor Books, pp.1-12.

GOFFMAN, E. (1972), *Encounters*, London Bobbs-Merrill.

GOULDNER, A.W. (1973), 'The Importance of Something for Nothing' in A.W. Gouldner, *For Sociology: Renewal and Critique in Sociology Today*, Harmondsworth, Penguin, pp.260-99.

HALL, E. (1959), *The Silent Language*, Garden City, Doubleday.

HALL, E. (1966), *The Hidden Dimension*, Garden City, Doubleday.

HENRY, J. (1972), *Culture against Man*, London, Random.

HORTON, J. (1967), 'Time and Cool People', *Trans-Action*, 4 (no.5), pp.5-12.

JOHNSON, M. (1975), 'Old Age and the Gift Relationship', *New Society*, vol.31, no.649, pp.639-42.

JOHNSON, S.K. (1971), *Idle Haven*, Berkeley, Los Angeles and London, University of California Press.

JUNG, C.G. (1971), 'The Stages of Life' in J. Campbell (ed.), *The Portable Jung*, New York, Viking.

KASTENBAUM, R. (1963), 'Cognitive and Personal Futurity in Later Life', *Journal of Individual Psychology*, 19, pp.216-22.

KIMMEL, D.C. (1974), *Adulthood and Aging*, New York, John Wiley.

KLUCKHOHN, F.R. (1953), 'Dominant and Variant Orientations' in C. Kluckhohn, H.A. Murray and D.H. Schneider (eds), *Personality in Nature, Society and Culture*, New York, Knopf.

KLUCKHOHN, F.R. and Strodtbeck, F.L. (1961), *Variations in Value Orientation*, New York, Harper & Row.

KUHLEN, R.G. (1964), 'Development Changes in Motivation During the Adult

Years' in J.E. Birren (ed.), *Relations of Development and Aging*, Springfield Illinois, Charles C. Thomas.

LEACH, E.R. (1966), 'Cronus and Chronos' in his *Rethinking Anthropology*, London, Athlone Press, pp.124-32.

LÉVI-STRAUSS, C. (1967), *The Savage Mind*, University of Chicago Press.

LIPMAN, V. (1959), *A Century of Social Services 1859-1959: The Jewish Board of Guardians*, London, Routledge & Kegan Paul.

MAGNUS, L. (1909), *The Jewish Board of Guardians and the Men Who Made It (1859-1909)*, London, Jewish Board of Guardians.

MALINOWSKI, B. (1927), 'Lunar and Seasonal Calendars in the Trobriands', *Journal of the Royal Anthropological Institute*, 57, pp.203-15.

MALTZ, D.N. (1968), 'Primitive Time Reckoning as a Symbolic System', *Cornell Journal of Social Relations*, 3, pp.85-111.

MAUSS, N. (1954), *The Gift*, London, Routledge & Kegan Paul.

MAXWELL, R.J. (1972), 'Anthropological Perspectives' in H. Yaker, H. Osmond and F. Cheek (eds), *The Future of Time*, New York, Anchor, pp. 36-72.

MEAD, G.H. (1964), 'Mind, Self and Society' in A. Strauss (ed.), *George Herbert Mead on Social Psychology*, University of Chicago Press.

MILLER, E.J. and GWYNNE, G.V. (1972), *A Life Apart*, London, Tavistock Publications.

NEUGARTEN, B.L. (1968), 'Adult Personality: Towards a Psychology of the Life Cycle' in E. Vinacke (ed.), *Reading in General Psychology*, New York, American Book Co.

NILSSON, M.P. (1920), *Primitive Time Reckoning*, Lund, C.W.K. Gleerup.

PECK, R.C. (1956), 'Psychological Developments in the Second Half of Life' in J.E. Anderson (ed.), *Psychological Aspects of Aging, Proceedings of the Conference on Planning Research, Bethesda Maryland April 24-27, 1955*, Washington DC, American Psychological Association.

RILEY, M.W. (1971), 'Social Gerontology and the Age Structure of Society', *Gerontologist*, 11, pp.79-87.

ROSENGREN, W.R. and LEFTON, M. (1969), *Hospitals and Patients*, New York, Atherton Press.

ROTH, J.A. (1963), *Timetables*, Indianopolis, Bobbs-Merrill.

SEELEY, J.R. *et al.*, (1956), *Crestwood Heights*, New York, Basic Books.

SIMMEL, G. (1964), 'Faithfulness and Gratitude' in K. Wolf (ed.), *The Sociology of Georg Simmel*, New York, Free Press.

SMITH, R.J. (1961), 'Cultural Differences in the Life Cycle and the Concepts of Time' in R.W. Klee (ed.), *Aging and Leisure*, New York, Oxford University Press, pp.83-103.

SMITH-BLAU, Z. (1973), *Old Age in a Changing Society*, New York, New View.

SOROKIN, P.A. and MERTON, R.K. (1937), 'Social Time: A Methodological and Functional Analysis', *American Journal of Sociology*, 42, pp.615-29.

STRAUSS, A. *et al.* (1963), 'The Hospital and its Negotiated Order' in E. Freidson (ed.), *The Hospital in Modern Society*, New York, The Free Press, pp. 147-69.

SYKES, G.M. (1966), *The Society of Captives: A Study of a Maximum Security Prison*, New York, Atheneum.

TITMUSS, R. (1973), *The Gift Relationship*, Harmondsworth, Penguin.

TOWNSEND, P. (1964), *The Last Refuge*, London, Routledge & Kegan Paul.

TOWNSEND, P. (1973), *The Family Life of Old People*, Harmondsworth, Penguin.

TURNER, V. (1967), *The Forest of Symbols*, Ithaca and London, Cornell University Press.

TURNER, V. (1969), *The Ritual Process*, London, Routledge & Kegan Paul,

WALLACE, S.E. (1971), 'On the Totality of Total Institutions' in his *Total Institutions* (ed.), USA, Transaction Books, pp. 1-8.

WISCHNITZER, M. (1948), *To Dwell in Safety*, Philadelphia, The Jewish Publication Society of America.

Index